Additional Titles for New Parents From the American Academy of Pediatrics

Baby and Toddler Basics: Expert Answers to Parents' Top 150 Questions

Baby Care Anywhere: A Quick Guide to Parenting On the Go

Caring for Your Baby and Young Child: Birth to Age 5*

Dad to Dad: Parenting Like a Pro

Food Fights: Winning the Nutritional Challenges of Parenthood Armed With Insight, Humor, and a Bottle of Ketchup

Guide to Toilet Training

Heading Home With Your Newborn: From Birth to Reality

Mama Doc Medicine: Finding Calm and Confidence in Parenting, Child Health, and Work-Life Balance

My Child Is Sick! Expert Advice for Managing Common Illnesses and Injuries

The New Baby Blueprint: Caring for You and Your Little One

New Mother's Guide to Breastfeeding

The Picky Eater Project: 6 Weeks to Happier, Healthier Family Mealtimes

Raising an Organized Child: 5 Steps to Boost Independence, Ease Frustration, and Promote Confidence

Raising Twins: Parenting Multiples From Pregnancy Through the School Years

Retro Baby: Cut Back on All the Gear and Boost Your Baby's Development With More Than 100 Time-tested Activities

Retro Toddler: More Than 100 Old-School Activities to Boost Development

Sleep: What Every Parent Needs to Know

Understanding the NICU: What Parents of Preemies and Other Hospitalized Newborns Need to Know

Your Baby's First Year*

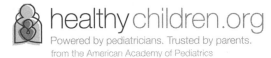

healthy children.org
Powered by pediatricians. Trusted by parents.
from the American Academy of Pediatrics

For additional parenting resources, visit the HealthyChildren bookstore at https://shop.aap.org/for-parents.

*This book is also available in Spanish.

The
CALM
Baby
Method

Solutions for Fussy Days
and Sleepless Nights

Patti Ideran, OTR/L, CEIM, and Mark Fishbein, MD, FAAP

American Academy of Pediatrics
DEDICATED TO THE HEALTH OF ALL CHILDREN®

American Academy of Pediatrics Publishing Staff

Mary Lou White, *Chief Product and Services Officer/SVP, Membership, Marketing, and Publishing*

Mark Grimes, *Vice President, Publishing*

Kathryn Sparks, *Senior Editor, Consumer Publishing*

Jason Crase, *Senior Manager, Production and Editorial Services*

Shannan Martin, *Production Manager, Consumer Publications*

Sara Hoerdeman, *Marketing Manager, Consumer Products*

Published by the American Academy of Pediatrics

345 Park Blvd

Itasca, IL 60143

Telephone: 630/626-6000

Facsimile: 847/434-8000

www.aap.org

The American Academy of Pediatrics is an organization of 67,000 primary care pediatricians, pediatric medical subspecialists, and pediatric surgical specialists dedicated to the health, safety, and well-being of all infants, children, adolescents, and young adults.

The information contained in this publication should not be used as a substitute for the medical care and advice of your pediatrician. There may be variations in treatment that your pediatrician may recommend based on individual facts and circumstances.

Statements and opinions expressed are those of the authors and not necessarily those of the American Academy of Pediatrics.

Any websites, brand names, products, or manufacturers are mentioned for informational and identification purposes only and do not imply an endorsement by the American Academy of Pediatrics (AAP). The AAP is not responsible for the content of external resources. Information was current at the time of publication.

The persons whose photographs are depicted in this publication are professional models. They have no relation to the issues discussed. Any characters they are portraying are fictional.

The publishers have made every effort to trace the copyright holders for borrowed materials. If they have inadvertently overlooked any, they will be pleased to make the necessary arrangements at the first opportunity.

This publication has been developed by the American Academy of Pediatrics. The contributors are expert authorities in the field of pediatrics. No commercial involvement of any kind has been solicited or accepted in development of the content of this publication. Disclosures: The authors report no financial disclosures.

Every effort is made to keep *The CALM Baby Method: Solutions for Fussy Days and Sleepless Nights* consistent with the most recent advice and information available from the American Academy of Pediatrics.

Special discounts are available for bulk purchases of this publication. Email Special Sales at nationalaccounts@aap.org for more information.

Printed in the United States of America

9-465/0321   1 2 3 4 5 6 7 8 9 10

CB0123

ISBN: 978-1-61002-482-2

eBook: 978-1-61002-485-3

EPUB: 978-1-61002-483-9

Kindle: 978-1-61002-484-6

Cover and publication design by Rattray Design

Library of Congress Control Number: 2020937622

What People Are Saying About
The CALM Baby Method

"*The CALM Baby Method: Solutions for Fussy Days and Sleepless Nights* should be the baby manual every new parent receives. Every page is full of immediately useful information, covering topics including reading infant cues, why babies cry, normal development, attachment, sleep, and soothing an upset baby. Reading this book will also calm distressed parents by putting practical tools in their hands."

> —Pec Indman, PA, EdD, MFT, PMH-C, coauthor of *Beyond the Blues: Understanding and Treating Prenatal and Postnatal Depression and Anxiety*

"If you are the parent of a newborn, this is the book to keep on your nightstand. *The CALM Baby Method: Solutions for Fussy Days and Sleepless Nights* is a valuable resource that provides practical and effective solutions to help parents feel confident when dealing with a fussy or high-needs baby. I enthusiastically recommend this book for all new parents!"

> —Anne H. Zachry, PhD, OTR/L, author of *Retro Baby* and associate professor and chair of occupational therapy, University of Tennessee Health Science Center

"A valuable and much-needed resource for parents and also professionals who work with infants and their families. Written in easy to understand language. Backed by years of experience from recognized experts. Parents of preemies and newborns will find many strategies to support a happier baby and positive successful feeding experiences. Professionals will appreciate the comprehensive information that is readily available to their practice."

> —Catherine S. Shaker, MS/CCC-SLP, BCS-S, senior clinician feeding and swallowing/NICU and pediatrics, AdventHealth for Children, https://shaker4swallowingandfeeding.com

"Colic is a complex phenomenon not easily addressed by simple strategies. In this book, Ideran and Fishbein have embraced that complexity in a clean and family-friendly way. This book provides insights into the multiple contributions to colic (including sensory, gastrointestinal, and social-emotional factors) while providing grounded suggestions of strategies to help families understand their own child's unique behavioral profile to individualize management of colic-related infant behavior."

> —Marie E. Anzalone, ScD, OTR/L, FAOTA, occupational therapist and coauthor of *Sensory Integration and Self-Regulation in Infants and Toddlers: Helping Very Young Children Interact With Their Environment*

"*The CALM Baby Method* is a wonderful resource full of practical advice and interventions to help parents understand their fussy baby. It empowers parents with the skills and confidence to calm their babies and gives them hope that happier days are ahead."

> —Michelle Jao, MD, FAAP, Northwestern Medicine Regional Medical Group

"The CALM approach is a practical, holistic way for parents to understand and soothe their fussy babies. Every parent can benefit from the strategies in this book!"

> —Lauren Little, PhD, OTR/L, associate professor of occupational therapy, Rush University

"I am honored to say I have a long and invigorating relationship with these authors. Their deeply grounded approach based on both evidence and decades of experience serving children and families is clear. They exemplify a collaborative interdisciplinary approach; families and professionals *must* have this book as a key reference."

> —Winnie Dunn, PhD, OTR, FAOTA, distinguished professor, occupational therapy, University of Missouri, and author of *Sensory Profile* assessments and *Living Sensationally: Understanding Your Senses*

"Dr Fishbein is a highly experienced pediatric gastroenterologist who has devoted his life to helping children and families. This book reflects his unique approach to caring for children and an entire career devoted to listening and learning."

—Miguel Saps, MD, professor of pediatrics, University of Miami Miller School of Medicine

"I had the pleasure of working with Dr Fishbein for 10 years as a member of our pediatric feeding team. He and Patti have written a great resource to help parents sort out what is a medical issue, a feeding problem, or colic. This book offers real-world intervention strategies for parents who are struggling, and it is a thorough and practical guide for families. A great resource."

—Cheri Fraker, MS, CCC/SLP, author of *Evaluation and Treatment of Pediatric Feeding Disorders: From NICU to Childhood* and coauthor of *Food Chaining: The Proven 6-Step Plan to Stop Picky Eating, Solve Feeding Problems, and Expand Your Child's Diet*

"This book is such a useful guide for families and pediatricians alike. It breaks down how to practically help infants learn the skills to self soothe and calm. So much of this book comes down to being present in the moment with the infant and engaging with the infant's cues. The tone in the book is full of respect for parents' ability to nurture. I wholeheartedly recommend *The CALM Baby Method: Solutions for Fussy Days and Sleepless Nights*."

—Kim Gehle, MD, FAAP, Northwestern Medicine

Equity, Diversity, and Inclusion Statement

The American Academy of Pediatrics is committed to principles of equity, diversity, and inclusion in its publishing program. Editorial boards, author selections, and author transitions (publication succession plans) are designed to include diverse voices that reflect society as a whole. Editor and author teams are encouraged to actively seek out diverse authors and reviewers at all stages of the editorial process. Publishing staff are committed to promoting equity, diversity, and inclusion in all aspects of publication writing, review, and production.

Authors and Contributors

Authors

Patti Ideran, OTR/L, CEIM
Chapters 1, 3, 4, 5, 6, 8, 9, 12, 14
Northwestern Medicine Central
 DuPage Hospital
Winfield, IL

Mark Fishbein, MD, FAAP
Chapter 2
Ann & Robert H. Lurie Children's
 Hospital of Chicago at
 Northwestern Medicine Central
 DuPage Hospital
Winfield, IL

Contributors

Kate Benton, PhD
Chapter 7
Ann & Robert H. Lurie Children's
 Hospital of Chicago at Northwestern
 Medicine Central DuPage Hospital
Winfield, IL

Diana Bohm, MS, CCC-SLP/L
Chapter 10
Northwestern Medicine Central
 DuPage Hospital
Winfield, IL

**Stephanie Krantz, RN, BSN, IBCLC,
PMH-C**
Chapter 13
Northwestern Medicine Central
 DuPage Hospital
Winfield, IL

Nicole Nalepa, RD, LDN
Chapter 11
Northwestern Medicine Central
 DuPage Hospital
Winfield, IL

Julie Stielstra, MLS
Contributing Editor
Northwestern Medicine Central
 DuPage Hospital
Winfield, IL

*To all the crying babies of the world (and the stressed parents),
you are being heard!*

Contents

Foreword

Andrea Childers, RN, BSN, CPN

As a pediatric nurse and mother of 2 teens and another tween, I understand that parenting is hard. The saying/adage, "The days are long, but the years are short," sticks out best to me in describing parenting. That quote has no meaning for parents with a colicky baby, though. Their days can't be so simply described as "long." Colicky babies can make the days seem unbearable. Parents want and need to know if it is possible to help make their challenges better.

Six years ago, I came to know and work with Mark Fishbein, MD, FAAP, in his pediatric gastroenterology clinic. Many a day, Dr Fishbein would come out of his initial assessment of a refluxing baby calling out, "We need Patti!" Patti Ideran, OTR/L, CEIM, has so much experience and insight on how to help babies experiencing challenges that Dr Fishbein would not want the family to leave until Patti could assure him they could be seen soon, as in *very* soon. He wanted to help the stressed baby and parents so that their medical concerns could then be properly assessed and help the parents learn how to calm and soothe their baby so that the fussiness might decrease. On those miracle days that Patti had no other patient conflict, she could come right in to meet the parents, and she would teach them how to better understand and respond to their babies. Parents would leave with a calmer baby and knowledge of what to do to help the next time their baby was colicky.

One such afternoon, a mother came to see Dr Fishbein with her 3-month-old son for an evaluation for reflux. Her baby was crying with no tears, wide-eyed, and thrashing his head. With frustration in her voice the mother explained she was there because "my baby has reflux so bad he never stops screaming." This was what we deemed a "we need Patti" moment. Thankfully, that day Patti was available to come. After an hour, I went to clean the room, presuming the mother had left after her appointment. She was still there holding her quiet, cooing son. Her frustration was gone, but she wasn't convinced he would stay calm. She and I reviewed the medical recommendations from

Dr Fishbein, as well as the calming strategies that Patti had given her. She was now able to head home equipped with resources and a community of people who wanted to help. A few days later I called her to check on them and heard a calm mother through the phone who wanted us to know that they were doing better.

Patti, along with Dr Fishbein and the other pediatric specialists who worked on this book, share what they have learned caring for babies and parents dealing with what is known as *colic*. We all hope to help make it better, because even though the medical books say colic may only last for a short time, each minute less makes those long hours a little shorter—and happier—for everyone.

Acknowledgments

This book was the brilliant idea of Andrea Childers, RN, BSN, CPN. As a nurse, she would see these colicky patients with Mark Fishbein, MD, FAAP; they would refer them to me; and she saw changes in both the babies and their parents and kept saying, "You should write this down." So, thank you, Andrea, for planting the seed—it is now written down!

A huge thank-you to Dr Fishbein and my fabulous team of authors. I have been fortunate enough to find a group of team members and coauthors who I deeply trust and have had the pleasure of working with for so many years. When you find a team like this, the sky is the limit. Specifically, I want to thank the following people for their individual talent:

- Kate Benton, PhD, for understanding and explaining behavior so eloquently to all of us and to the parents we work with.
- Nicole Nalepa, RD, LDN, for helping so many parents feel better about their babies' nutrition (and for naming me the "baby whisperer"—it really stuck!).
- Julie Stielstra, MLS, for your many edits and finding everything I needed on the topic; I would say, "Sounds like…," and you would find it!
- Stephanie Krantz, RN, BSN, IBCLC, PMH-C, for your boundless energy and your shared passion with me of babies and their mommies.
- Diana Bohm, MS, CCC-SLP/L, for your quiet excellence. I observe you listening and watching these babies, and you are in a zone assessing the quality of their suck, swallow, and breathe synchrony—and you are always right!
- Dr Fishbein, you are so smart (as we all say), and we have learned so much from you. Thanks for guiding our team to keep reaching new heights, and thanks for pushing me (respectfully) to write this book.

I am deeply grateful to my mentors, experts in their fields. Some I had the pleasure of knowing: Winnie Dunn, PhD, OTR, FAOTA; Zack Boukydis, PhD; Jodi Mindell, PhD, CBSM; and Megan Faure, BSc, OT, OTR, your passion for the work you do shines within me. Some mentors who I have read and studied have molded my knowledge and passion about the subject of infants: T. Berry Brazelton, MD; J. Kevin Nugent, PhD; Mechthild Papousek, MD, Prof; Ian St. James-Roberts, PhD, FBPsS; and Georgia DeGangi, PhD, OTR, FAOTA.

Thanks to my baby models in the book and their parents: Addilyn (Chrissy and Corey), Aurora (Jen and Mark), Ellliot (Melissa and Eric), Jay (Erica and John), Noah (Steven and Lindsay), Norah (Erin and Joe), Orson (Kassi and Trey), and Owen (Ariel and Nick). I hope you had fun doing the baby yoga poses and baby massage. Always hug and play with your babies; they grow up so fast!

I appreciate all the support from my many colleagues over the years who referred to me, supported me, advised me, challenged me with questions, and understood my passion for these fussy babies; so many to name, but especially Laura Colucci, RN, BSN; Michelle Jao, MD, FAAP; Kristen Vogt, MD, FAAP; Liz Maryuama, MPH, OTR; Jenn Zieman, MOT, OTR/L, CEIM; Kelly Brown, MOT, OTR/L, CEIM; Jessica Kronberg, MOT, OTR/L; Amy Wolfinger, PT, CEIM; Kassi Hemming, PT, DPT, CIMI; Linda Hammond, PT, DPT; and Jesse Coffelt, PT, DPT.

Thanks to the thousands of babies and their parents who have allowed me to be in their lives; you have helped me learn even more about babies and the challenges families face during this demanding time. I run into you every once in a while, and it is always so rewarding that you still remember how much it helped early on!

I appreciate all my many close friends and family members (especially Carol Garrison, Sandy Jelm, Barb Thompson, and Jen Perniciaro) who supported me along this journey. I know my parents (Dean and Janie Weeks) and my friend Lisa Dapas are smiling down from above.

Finally, my immediate family. I'm extremely proud of both my boys, Steven and Gregory. Parenting you boys has made me a better person. I am eternally blessed that I had the pleasure of raising you; parenting is hard work—but you made it easy. I am indebted to my wonderful husband, Dave, who believed in me when I wasn't always sure. During this project you did more cooking, gave me a shoulder rub when I was on the computer too long, and brought me a glass of wine to help me change gears. You are a rock, and nothing I have accomplished in my life would have been possible without you.

Patti Ideran, OTR/L, CEIM

I wish to acknowledge my fellow members of our pediatric feeding disorders team: Nicole Nalepa, RD, LDN; Kate Benton, PhD; Diana Bohm, MS, CCC-SLP/L; Laura Colucci, RN, BSN; Patti Ideran, OTR/L, CEIM; and Andrea Childers, RN, BSN, CPN, for whose knowledge, devotion, and passion have made this book possible. I would also like to extend my gratitude to my wife, Margie, and children, Katie, Ellie, Joey, and Tricia, for always being there for me. Finally, I would like to thank my instructors, peers, and patients for providing me with insight and giving me the opportunity to share the knowledge that I have acquired all these years.

Mark Fishbein, MD, FAAP

Introduction
Patti Ideran, OTR/L, CEIM

Having a baby is a thrilling experience. Having a fussy or high-need baby…
well, it can be a challenge! Ask any parent who has ever had a fussy baby
what it's like and we all remember vividly, no matter how long ago it was. My
first baby was an angel. He ate well, slept well, was always happy and content, and fussed only a little when he was hungry. I was tired, but I thought,
"This is easy!" I never questioned my parenting skills on my first baby. It
is very rewarding as a mom to be able to calm your baby but extremely
discouraging when you cannot. This is the fussy baby, my second baby. I
second-guessed myself all the time on my fussy/high-need baby. The questions were nonstop: What could be wrong with my baby? What was I doing
wrong? How could I emotionally deal with a fussy baby? And would I ever
get a good night's sleep again? I often felt lost on how to parent this beautiful
but fussy baby. I felt inadequate to help him through his irritability. I did
get through it, with the support of my great husband and family. And my
fussy baby did grow out of it and was a fabulous toddler. That experience led
me to devote my time and energy to understanding and addressing these
types of babies. I first started helping friends and my clients to understand
their fussy or irritable babies. This was also when I met Mark Fishbein, MD,
FAAP, pediatric gastroenterologist, my mentor and the driving force behind
writing this book. We had many discussions about babies with colic and
how we could help them and their parents. He would evaluate the medical
causes and I would work on the behavioral piece. And it worked! During
this period, 91% of our referrals for infant colic showed almost immediate
improvement in either fussiness, sleeping, or feeding.

In today's climate of TMI (too much information), it can feel overwhelming when you try to look online and learn about your fussy baby. There are
many "mommy blogs" or social media posts and messages with inaccurate,
unreliable, or even harmful advice. You probably also receive all sorts of
loving tips from well-meaning grandparents, friends, or sisters…but if they

have not parented a fussy baby themselves, they can't truly understand what you are going through. You've probably also made many calls and visits to your pediatrician's office, and your doctor suggests a variety of solutions, although none of them seem to work and often you don't feel heard. Then all this advice starts to conflict and contradict…it's overwhelming. Babies may be labeled as being colicky or high need or sensitive or unsettled or immature or fussy…they really all mean the same thing. You will hear that they will grow out of it at about 3 or 4 months—but you need help now with your baby's fussy days and sleepless nights.

That is why we wrote this book. We wrote it to introduce you to the CALM Baby Method: *c*ues, *a*rousal *l*evels, and *m*assage. In the following chapters, you learn about

- **Cues:** Because babies can't tell you how they feel, they communicate with you through their behaviors, or *cues*. They tell you, "I'm tired," or "I'm hungry." It is important to understand that fussy babies often do not give clear cues, which can make it difficult to know what they want. Learning to read your baby's cues helps to decrease your stress and improve your confidence in yourself as a parent.
- **Arousal *levels*** or **behavioral states of arousal:** This describes how alert or how sleepy your baby is at different times, and you learn how this affects how you care for your baby. You learn to recognize specific, predictable (or sometimes unpredictable!) states of alertness in your baby.
- ***Massage:*** This book incorporates the importance of human touch and massage. Babies of this generation are sometimes called "container babies." They are in bouncy seats, swings, or carriers and are being held and touched much less than maybe you were as a baby. Too much use of this equipment has contributed to mild developmental delays, flat heads, and less bonding between baby and parent. In this book, we talk about the importance of getting your baby *out* of these pieces of equipment and give you positioning suggestions, which also helps with your baby's motor development.

Other topics in the book include

- **What is colic?** We help you understand what colic is and tease out the symptoms that could be related to medical issues (eg, gastrointestinal issues, feeding problems, immaturity) or behavioral issues (eg, state regulation, poor sleep, a tendency toward overstimulation).

- **Your baby's sensory world:** Our philosophy about fussy babies is that they are often overstimulated by the outside world, and that can be exhausting! Overstimulation affects your baby's entire personality. In a later chapter, you will learn about what your baby experiences through her senses, her crying behaviors, and how her sleep (or lack of sleep) affects her behavior.
- **Attachment:** The content on attachment teaches you what attachment is and how it can be difficult with a fussy or high-need baby. You will be provided information on infant attachment, why it is important, how attachments develop, and how they are maintained.
- **Sleep:** In this book, we address the importance of sleep, safe sleep practices, and typical sleep patterns in babies, as well as the challenges fussy babies have with sleep. We also detail sleep training and creating a conducive sleep environment to help your baby *and* you receive some well-needed sleep.
- **Feeding and nutrition:** This content covers what typical feeding is and what to do when there are problems. You will also learn about all the different nutritional interventions on the market these days for fussy babies and the research behind them.
- **"Baby blues":** Postpartum depression can be made worse when you have a fussy baby. We give you information on this important issue and talk about how it can affect the whole family.
- **Beyond colic:** What if your baby is still colicky after the typical age? We help you understand some of your baby's unique issues and where to go for help.

We have helped thousands of parents just like you with babies like your own. We wrote this book to help you and your fussy baby. (My former fussy baby is now a wonderfully successful, happy young adult. He likes to take credit for my career path—and he's right. Thanks, Greg!)

The CALM Baby Method: Solutions for Fussy Days and Sleepless Nights helps you become an expert at understanding your baby and can give you a calmer, happier baby. And then *you* will be calmer, happier, and ready to adore your little bundle of joy.

Chapter 1

What Is Colic?

What is colic? That is the million-dollar question! If you are reading about colic maybe you have a fussy baby or a fussy grandbaby or a friend who is dealing with a fussy baby. You may even just be an expecting parent wanting to learn more about babies. The content in this chapter gives you the most recent updated information on colic and common symptoms that may indicate a baby is experiencing colic. *Colic* is not really an actual disease or diagnosis—the discomfort, the crying, and the fussiness are a collection of symptoms that occur together in a pattern. Sometimes doctors and nurses don't even like to say the word "colic" because they know the word is dreaded by parents. They know parents have read all the baby books and have hoped and prayed their baby wouldn't have it. Instead of saying "colic," doctors may choose alternate words to describe your baby; they may say you have a *high-need* baby, a *sensitive* baby, an *unsettled* baby, a baby who cries excessively for no apparent reason, an *inconsolable* baby, an *irritable* baby, a baby who is just on the immature side, or a baby with a difficult temperament. That is what I (Patti) was told back when my son was a baby. When I asked, "How is this different than colic?" they said it wasn't. Bottom line: *colic* is merely a label that covers the range of symptoms and possible causes. And for you, as a parent, that word tells you there will be some challenging times ahead. Colic is very overwhelming to families; it may cause strained relationships between parents, between baby and parents, even between parents and *their* parents. Inconsistent and sometimes unpredictable crying is a hallmark of colic, and this crying affects many things. It can disrupt lives, feed into social isolation, and make parents desperately search for a medical diagnosis. It can also make postpartum depression worse. (Read more about the postpartum family in Chapter 13.) It is the primary reason for phone calls to the pediatrician during a baby's first 6 months. Because there is not a proven treatment, parents can often be frustrated with no solid answer as to *why* their baby is crying so much.

Sound Familiar?

Here are some common concerns about fussy babies parents share with pediatricians.

- She's super sensitive.
- I can't put him down.
- This baby is draining.
- She's unpredictable and unsatisfied.
- He doesn't like to cuddle, which breaks my heart.
- He is intense.
- She seems hyperactive.
- She wants to nurse *all the time.*
- My baby is demanding.
- She awakens frequently and doesn't seem to be well rested.

What Is Colic?

The definition is vague and varied. The "classic" definition of colic (around since the 1950s!) is the sudden onset of high-pitched crying without a medical reason in an otherwise healthy, well-fed baby that happens for 3 hours per day, for more than 3 days per week, for more than 3 weeks (the *rule of 3s*). So that means your baby will have colic for at least 3 weeks before your pediatrician will even call it colic! Current information from the scientific literature in medicine and psychology has resulted in additions to that definition over the years, which may now include:

- Crying 3 hours per day for 3 or more days per week for 1 week (vs 3 weeks in the original definition).
- Not calming when picked up; attempts at soothing them often result in babies stiffening or arching the body with no settling. The usual soothing strategies, such as holding, rocking, or listening to mother's voice, are not effective.

❧ A disturbance in the sleep-wake cycle; they often have very short sleep phases during the day. They are frequently called *cat-nappers*.

❧ Difficulties getting to sleep and staying asleep; it takes a long time to finally settle them to sleep, and then they wake and you have to try again. They often sleep fewer hours than typical babies per day.

❧ Difficulties falling and staying in deep sleep. Parents have described them as restless sleepers; parents need to keep the house *very* quiet because any little noise wakes them. Fussy babies often wake more frequently than typical babies.

❧ Difficulties self-regulating their states of arousal (ie, deep sleep, light sleep, quiet alert, active alert, fussing, crying). These babies do not move through all levels easily or they stay primarily in one—crying!

❧ Crying episodes such as intense crying, quickly escalating from 0 to 60 in no time; nonspecific crying; or feeding-related crying.

❧ Unable to feed properly, although they don't usually have difficulty gaining weight. They are on and off the nipple during a feeding, distracted easily during feeding, and sometimes feed too often.

❧ Overly alert, they are often called *hyperalert* or *wide-eyed* or are said to have a "hunger for stimulation." Parents often equate this to not needing sleep; however, these babies are usually overtired and need sleep but look hyperalert.

❧ Difficulty regulating responses to everyday stimuli; they overreact to stimuli such as a dog barking, a door slamming, being moved, or having a diaper change and often have difficulty recovering from these stimuli.

Did You Know?

Certified lactation consultants are specialists in breastfeeding who can help mothers learn how to successfully breastfeed their babies. Sometimes the fussiness babies exhibit may not be colic but may stem from problems with breastfeeding. These issues include milk supply (low or overabundant supply), overactive letdown reflex, or improper latch. If you are having difficulties with breastfeeding, make an appointment with a lactation consultant through your local hospital. (See Chapter 10 for more information).

Colic Characteristics

How common is colic? It occurs in anywhere from 10% to 40% of babies. It is equally distributed across races and socioeconomic statuses and between boys and girls. Whether you breastfeed or bottle-feed does not seem to increase or decrease the chances of your baby having colic. There is no grading of colic, such as mild, moderate, or severe. However, it is clear that colic is not caused by a disease or anything a parent has done. This is very important for parents to understand. Colic can occur in spite of excellent parenting. The "classic colic curve" starts at about 1 to 2 weeks of age, peaks at 6 to 8 weeks of age, and drops off by 14 to 16 weeks of age. Often, most of the crying happens in the early evening, but some babies cry all day long (or it seems like it!). Sometimes the intensity of the crying is stronger in the early evening.

Is Colic More Prevalent in Other Countries?

Several years ago, there was a review of studies that looked at the incidence of colic in 8 countries: United States, Denmark, Germany, Japan, Canada, United Kingdom, the Netherlands, and Italy. The most consistent finding was a lower fuss or cry duration in Denmark, with the Netherlands and Canada having significantly higher fuss or cry duration. Researchers could only speculate on the reasons why, such as economic conditions, caregiving patterns, baby wearing or carrying (less equipment), and feeding style. These studies should be interpreted cautiously, as many variables were not measured and many countries were not included, but studies such as these may help us eventually understand colic more. (This doesn't mean if you move to Denmark, your baby won't have colic!)

Not all fussy babies show all characteristics or symptoms, but most do show several of them. Typical babies may show some of these symptoms; however, it is the intensity and duration that separates a "typical" baby from a "colicky" baby. Crying in a colicky baby is more persistent and severe than in typical babies. A true diagnosis of colic is not only a cry complaint but includes some of the other symptoms listed previously. When do the symptoms lead to diagnosing colic? It is diagnosed when the symptoms cause impairment or dysfunction with the baby (eg, poor feeding, poor sleep, increased irritability) or distress in the family (eg, attachment, parental stress, relationship difficulties between the parents, postpartum depression). A classic consequence of colic is that parents often revert to dysfunctional strategies (understandably) because nothing has worked! They hold their baby, stroll with them, drive them around at all hours, and feed them nonstop.

Excessive crying is one of the most common problems in the first year after birth and probably the least understood. We know that colic does end, but you may be told it is not harmful to your baby, it is trivial, and they will grow out of it. Explanations that colic is harmless or trivial are not helpful to overstressed parents whose lives revolve around caring for their fussy baby around the clock. Colic is a *huge* challenge for parents! Empathy from anyone, including health care professionals, doesn't offer the structured concrete strategies needed, such as the ones discussed in this book. Research has shown that colic causes tremendous distress in the baby-mother relationship and should not be overlooked. There is an increased cost to the health care system as parents search for explanations and answers for their baby's crying. There may be multiple visits (or phone calls) to their doctor and even trips to the emergency department for excessive crying—only to be discharged with no explanation.

In the scientific literature from the medical and psychological worlds, there are generally 4 different viewpoints on the possible causes of colic. What is known is that there is *not* a consensus on what colic is. These viewpoints include the following areas:

1. A gastrointestinal issue, or a stomach or intestinal explanation, such as gas, acid reflux, tummy pain, esophagitis, low-grade systemic inflammation, or swallowing air during crying (*aerophagia*).
2. An immature nervous system, causing overreaction to stimuli, disorganized responses, unpredictable cues, feeding difficulties, or poor sleep patterns.
3. Possible allergies or intolerance to cow's milk protein in the diet of breastfeeding mothers.
4. Some theorists even describe parenting behavior as an explanation; however, as previously explained, it is clear that colic is not caused by anything a parent has done. Health care professionals sometimes attribute colic to first-time, inexperienced, or anxious parents; however, research disputes this. On rare occasions colic can occur in homes with environmental tension, neglect, or mental health issues with family members.

Other, less obvious explanations in pediatric literature linked to colic are maternal smoking while pregnant, low birth weight, restlessness of the baby, or mother's distress during pregnancy. These explanations vary widely.

Some babies who are diagnosed with colic have none of these issues, and some babies with colic may have more than one. Bottom line is that we want babies who have colic to be identified so we can eliminate the risks and consequences of colic and provide supportive treatment to families. What we don't want to happen is for these babies to be labeled as "difficult" early in their lives, as this leads to parental helplessness and may lead to parents feeling their baby will "always" be difficult. We need to listen to parents and give them support, guidance, and assistance.

Did You Know?

There was a large study out of Denmark that looked at the risk of colic in preterm babies and babies that were considered small for gestational age. This is when a baby is born term but is smaller than most babies that are born term and are usually under the 10th percentile. The study found that these preterm and small babies were at increased risk of developing colic. They found there was a 30% chance of these babies developing colic if they were born before 37 weeks of gestation. They also found that the risk increased the earlier they were born, with the highest odds when babies were born at 32 weeks of gestation. If you have a preterm baby or a baby who is small for gestational age and your baby also has colic, consider an evaluation by an occupational therapist who is experienced in working with preterm babies and fussy babies. The sooner you intervene, the more positive outcomes you will have.

Source: Milidou I, Søndergaard C, Jensen MS, Olsen J, Henriksen TB. Gestational age, small for gestational age, and infantile colic. *Paediatr Perinat Epidemiol.* 2014;28(2):138–145.

Risks and Consequences of Colic

Parents of fussy babies are often exhausted and harbor feelings of guilt and helplessness—and sometimes anger. What we do know is that babies who cry excessively are at a higher risk for child abuse and neglect or even shaken baby syndrome. (See the "Child Abuse Is Preventable" box in Chapter 3.) Some abuse to children is called *abusive head trauma*, which is caused by striking, blunt object impact, throwing, or dropping a baby. Shaken baby syndrome is a subset of abusive head trauma. Abuse to fussy babies can also lead to fractures and bruises. Excessive crying can often lead to parents losing patience. This can happen with some well-meaning caregivers, who are just at the breaking point with their crying baby. Make sure you get help and support from family and friends—you need a break sometimes!

Where the AAP Stands: Abusive Head Trauma

The term *abusive head trauma* was adopted by the American Academy of Pediatrics (AAP) in 2009 in recognition of the fact that inflicted head injury of children can involve a variety of biomechanical forces, including but not limited to shaking. Shaking typically refers to the baby picked up around the chest and shaken back and forth, causing the head to whiplash back and forth. This change in terminology from shaken baby syndrome to abusive head trauma, however, was misinterpreted by some in the legal and medical communities as an indication of some doubt in or invalidation of the diagnosis and the mechanism of shaking as a cause of injury. The AAP continues to affirm the dangers and harms of shaking babies and continues to embrace the shaken baby syndrome diagnosis as a valid subset of an abusive head trauma diagnosis. Education is key in the prevention of this devastating injury. This includes educating anyone who has contact with your baby (eg, child care, babysitters, other family members). The AAP encourages pediatric practitioners to educate community stakeholders when necessary.

Source: Narang SK, Fingarson A, Lukefahr J; American Academy of Pediatrics Council on Child Abuse and Neglect. Abusive head trauma in infants and children. *Pediatrics*. 2020;145(4):e20200203.

There are other consequences to having a fussy baby. It can interfere with forming a strong bond between a baby and the parents (refer to Chapter 7 on attachment). Often, moms are the only one who can best calm a fussy baby, usually because they can breastfeed, and fathers or partners sometimes take a back seat in the care. This can allow the partner to care for other siblings, but it means they often miss out on intimate bonding moments with the baby. Having a fussy baby also can affect the relationship between the mother and other siblings; attending to the fussy baby all day long limits the time spent with her other children. This can easily feed into a mother's anxiety and lead to postpartum depression. (Refer to Chapter 13 for more information on postpartum depression.)

Another risk of having a fussy baby is premature cessation of breastfeeding, as the baby may not be feeding well (see Chapter 10). This often happens because the breastfeeding problems are not identified or corrected early enough and mothers give up and discontinue breastfeeding. Breastfeeding is best during the first year after birth; if it must be discontinued because of various reasons, it can be frustrating and emotionally devastating for some moms. Some moms have the dream or goal of breastfeeding their baby throughout the first year, and when this doesn't happen it can directly affect a mother's emotional well-being. We always recommend working with a lactation consultant first before making the decision to cease breastfeeding.

Another risk of colic is that sometimes a fussy baby can be overfed. This happens because fussy babies can't calm on their own and often can only calm when being nursed or bottle-fed. In these cases, babies suck/eat to calm, not for hunger, leading to poor establishment of hunger and satiation (fullness) cycles. Sometimes overfeeding makes colic worse, as babies can become uncomfortable, more irritable, or have increased burping and spitting up, and this becomes a negative cycle.

There is a lack of scientific evidence to explain the reasons for colic, so there is no standard, proven treatment available that all physicians use or recommend. Often, strategies are subjective for each baby and situation. We know how frustrating it can be for parents to not be able to get solid answers for why their baby cries so desperately. Unfortunately, because there is no standard treatment or conclusive answers as to why babies are crying, recommendations are often piecemeal and advice can be inconsistent. Because there is a lack of understanding as to what causes colic, there is a lack of consistent management strategies.

Did You Know?

Researchers in Australia are discussing the benefits of an integrated or coordinated approach to treat colic. This approach would start in the early weeks of fussiness with a treatment strategy that would focus on both the parents and the baby. It would include medical support from pediatricians and gastrointestinal doctors and nurses, lactation support to reduce the risk of ceasing breastfeeding, and support from speech therapists to assist with feeding difficulties. Emotional support is provided to the parents through counseling, support groups, or parent-to-parent help. Occupational therapists would start treating these babies early, looking at developmental, behavioral, and social-emotional issues, and provide needed environmental modifications early.

Source: Douglas PS, Mares RE, Hill PS. Interdisciplinary perspectives on the management of the unsettled baby: key strategies for improved outcomes. *Aust J Prim Health.* 2012;18(4):332–338.

Our goal with this book is to educate parents about our approach to colic using the CALM Baby Method. The solutions in this book are suggestions that look at the "whole" baby and their families. There is no guarantee that there is one solution that can help you and your fussy baby, but with education and the use of the CALM Baby Method, we hope to help reduce your baby's crying and improve your baby's sleep and feeding issues and help you get through this overwhelming time!

"I realized that colic was just a word. One doctor said it was colic; another said he was just a high-need baby; but he was still just my baby. What I learned is that there are strategies to help and I don't have to wait for him to grow out of it!"

Mother of a 2-month-old fussy baby

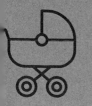

Chapter 2

Is It Colic or Something Else?

Having a baby who cries excessively is overwhelming, distressing, and worrisome for all parents. As you will learn in Chapter 3, there are many different cries, but when a baby is considered to have excessive crying, you need to find out what is going on. Babies with colic or excessive crying have distinct features in their crying and body language. Physicians describe crying in colic as louder and higher pitched. It may sound as if babies are in pain because it is more intense—and they are *screaming!* Physicians have described distinct symptoms of what colic looks like and what parents see, including

- Inconsolable cry with concurrent clenching of the fists with flexion of the hips.
- Clenching of the fists and flexion of the hips suggestive of abdominal discomfort.

The first person to whom you should mention this crying concern is your primary care physician, but sometimes your first opportunity to mention it is to an emergency department physician. First, the doctor will do a thorough intake (history) and general examination. Your baby will be checked for other possible problems that may contribute to excessive crying, even uncommon ones. Some of the diagnoses your primary care physician will rule out include ear infection (otitis media), urinary tract infection, or even meningitis. There also could be an accidental trauma to your baby that causes pain and excessive crying, such as a corneal abrasion (ie, a scratch on the eye), foreign body in the eye, hair tourniquet (this is when a piece of hair gets wrapped around the finger, toe, or even the penis), bug bite, or fractured clavicle. The major gastrointestinal disorders that are often attributed to colic include gastroesophageal reflux and food allergy (both discussed later in this chapter) and lactose intolerance. In most instances, these diagnoses are not applicable to the colicky baby and are falsely identified and targeted. A medical diagnosis is applicable in only 5% of cases.

At each of your baby's well-child (health supervision) visit appointments, as well as during a sick visit, your baby's height (length), weight, and head circumference will be measured and recorded. These routine measurements track your baby's growth and provide your doctor with an indication of appropriate weight gain or possible concern of weight loss. The head circumference provides a measure to determine whether the skull and brain are growing in proportion to your baby's size. Figure 2.1 is a sample growth chart of a baby girl, showing length and weight measurements for 4 clinic visits between the ages 1 and 6 months.

Individual growth charts for both boys and girls are designed to apply to all sized babies and are used to determine adequate progression. (See Resources for examples of growth charts for length, weight, and head circumference.) Babies with colic typically do not have problems with weight gain, but it is standard practice to always check weight, height, and head circumference. Similar charting of your baby's length and head circumference is done at your pediatrician's office for each well-child visit.

You will be asked about your pregnancy, including whether there were any complications, how long it was, what kind of delivery you had, your baby's birth weight, and how long you and your baby stayed in the hospital after birth. Family history is also important. Any genetic or familial disorders and the health of your other children or family members should be told to your doctor.

The doctor will also want to know about your baby's feeding, breast or bottle; if bottle-fed, what type of formula; how often, how much, how well, and how long your baby eats; and whether your baby vomits or spits up after feeding. See Chapter 10 for more information on feeding skills in your baby and what kinds of issues should be brought up to your pediatrician.

Your primary care physician will also make note of your baby's general development and behavior, including head movements and control; ability to move arms and legs and grasp things; ability to see, hear, and respond to sudden noises (startle response); strength of crying; and general strength and muscle tone. Low tone (tending toward floppiness) or high tone (tending toward stiffness) is important to note during the physical examination, as it may influence development. *Developmental delay* means that a child has not achieved appropriate milestones for his or her age. There is variability in the degree of developmental delay that a child may possess, and any identified delays will need to be

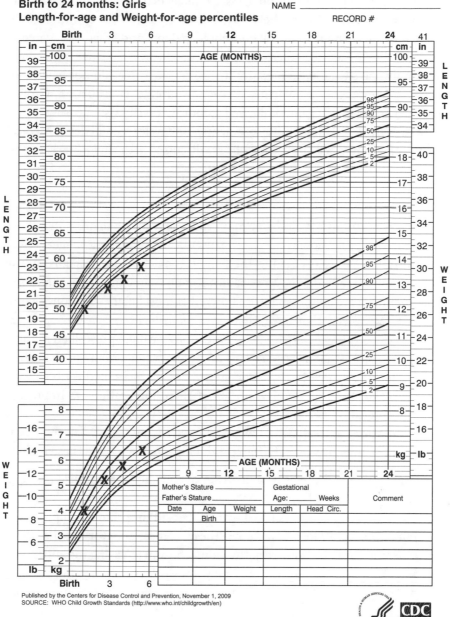

Figure 2.1. The growth chart depicts 4 clinic visits between ages 1 and 6 months with normal weight gain and growth for an infant girl. This child is following the 25th percentile for weight and second percentile for length. The head circumference is also measured at each visit but is depicted in a separate growth chart. A comparable growth chart is used for infant boys.

tracked over time to determine progress. Examples of developmental delay in an infant may include inability to hold up the head or track an object with the eyes.

Other information about the household, parents, and other adult caregivers in the home may be gathered as well so the doctor can better understand the family and situation. In most instances, colicky babies do not have associated symptoms such as diarrhea, extreme vomiting, constipation, swollen abdomen, poor weight gain, prolonged jaundice (ie, yellowish coloring visible in skin, eyes, etc, relating to liver problems), or developmental delay. Medical disorders that have been linked to colic are discussed in the following sections.

GERD and GER

Because we can't always find a specific cause for colicky distress in babies, some medical professionals may associate colic with gastroesophageal reflux disease (GERD)—excess acid in the baby's stomach and esophagus. In the first few months after birth, most babies spit up frequently, regurgitate, and may vomit, but recent research has shown that most babies with colic do not have GERD; instead, they have what we call *uncomplicated gastroesophageal reflux* (GER). Although anti-reflux medications are often prescribed in these instances, they are not necessary and do not help colic. Many of the babies that I (Dr Fishbein) see in my clinic are already on these medications (with little success); therefore, education about these medications is important and encouraged.

Medications to treat GERD work by neutralizing the acid in the stomach or by keeping the stomach from producing too much acid. These include

- Antacids (eg, Maalox, Mylanta). They act quickly to neutralize the acid so it is less harmful.
- Histamine (H_2) blockers (eg, Tagamet, Pepcid) or proton pump inhibitors (eg, Prilosec, Nexium). These medications work in slightly different ways, but both keep the stomach from releasing too much acid. H_2 blockers are milder and may not work as well over time as proton pump inhibitors. Both of these medications are safe and can be bought over the counter, with rare side effects.

Gastroesophageal reflux is a common problem in all babies; most younger babies have it to some degree. Reflux may be present in up to 80% of babies and is more common in preterm babies. The esophageal sphincter, the valve between the esophagus and the entrance to the stomach, may open up at the wrong time in babies and, thus, allow the stomach contents to come back into the esophagus (reflux). The amount and timing may vary as an infant grows, but generally most babies tolerate reflux without any problem. In fact, these babies are often called "happy spitters," because they seem otherwise comfortable and eat and grow well. As babies grow older, generally by 6 to 12 months of age, the esophageal sphincter should open in a more appropriate fashion and keep the stomach contents where they belong. These babies probably do not require any diagnostic testing or medication. Reassurance is provided and standard reflux precautions are offered. These precautions include

- Keeping your baby upright after feeding for 20 to 30 minutes, preferably by holding your baby.
- Avoiding baby seats or swings right after eating. These positions tend to place unwanted pressure on the belly and make symptoms of reflux worse.
- Avoiding excessive use of baby equipment (see Chapter 12), as it may worsen symptoms.

Did You Know?

Thickening the feeds with rice cereal or oatmeal is sometimes recommended to help keep formula down; however, this treatment has not been proven to help with reflux. It is important to remember that thickening the formula flow (out of the nipple) may cause your baby to work harder to feed—perhaps *too* hard. Therefore, care must be taken in these instances, and you may find that thickening is not worthwhile. A pre-thickened formula may be more appealing for babies with spitting up because it does not thicken until reaching the stomach.

Allergies or Protein Sensitivity

It is important to note what symptoms a baby shows when she is "colicky." As mentioned previously, spitting up or occasional, random vomiting is common and does not necessarily contribute to colic. However, there may be symptoms that are associated with a baby's feeding or taking milk, and these other possibilities should be investigated. For example, there could be an allergy or sensitivity to the proteins in human or cow's milk.

Human and cow's milk contain similar proteins. There is also soy formula, based on proteins made from soy. However, babies allergic to cow's or human milk might also react to soy milk. Reactions to these proteins might be mild or quite severe, ranging from hives or a rash around the mouth to vomiting and diarrhea. Changing the milk source might stop the problem. There are also low-allergy formulas, made with proteins that have already been partially broken down or digested, so they cause less reaction in sensitive babies and can help quite quickly. Such an allergy or sensitivity to milk proteins might be related to colic, but it is important to watch for other symptoms and when they occur. In more severe cases, you may need to carefully try different foods or milk for different lengths of time to figure out what works best and safely. When no other formula can be used safely, elemental formula, which contains only amino acids instead of intact proteins, may be prescribed. Elemental formula is not indicated for the colicky baby without any overt symptoms such as rash, vomiting, or diarrhea. All these special formulas contain all the nutrients that a baby needs to grow. But because breastfeeding is the best source of nutrition for you baby during the first year, it is very important to continue breastfeeding if possible (see Chapter 11).

What Can Be Done

The natural history of colic is well known to primary care physicians. They are aware that colic is self-limited and that within a few months your baby will have outgrown the condition. Therefore, aside from changing the baby formula or perhaps treating with anti-reflux medication, they generally may provide reassurance and send you on your way. But there is so much more that can be done to help your fussy baby. In my practice, over the years, I have learned that these babies almost immediately benefit, in the proper setting, from consultations with an occupational therapist and/or speech therapist for calming and swallow evaluation, respectively.

My responsibility is to determine whether fussiness is derived from a medical condition, as previously discussed in this chapter, or, more likely, a baby's inability to calm or swallow properly—or perhaps a combination of both. Important clues discussed in later chapters include whether a baby is hyperalert, overstimulated, hypervigilant, fidgety, having poor state control, or demanding constant attention. These behaviors are draining on parents! I also note whether babies are difficult to feed, have prolonged feeding sessions, are in distress during feedings, and have audible (loud, gulpy) swallows. Babies who were born preterm or who have developmental delay are at greatest risk for fussiness and feeding difficulties, but these problems are not exclusive to them. Of particular interest are babies who we expect to be swallowing excessive air during feedings. Air swallowing is the particular reason that babies are burped. Gas drops are often provided to fussy babies to counteract their gassiness (after the fact), but a more effective approach is to prevent excessive air swallowing as it occurs. Prevention of excessive air swallowing during feeds is discussed in Chapter 10.

Addressing Colicky Babies

Full-term babies from uncomplicated pregnancies are also at risk of colic, which may be more of a surprise to parents. I have found that the road less traveled is to discuss my concerns with the caregivers and provide detailed information concerning the rationale for my referrals to an occupational therapist and/or speech therapist. The temptation is to always go with the quick fix, including a change of formula or adding anti-reflux medication, but neither is truly helpful in this situation (if they were, perhaps there would not be any need to write this book). Yet seeing is believing, and for many of my referrals, patient and parent satisfaction are quite high. There are no magic tricks or illusions to helping colicky babies, only proper insight and care that will yield the results that your baby deserves.

Over time, I am hopeful that other physicians adapt a similar triage process in addressing colicky babies and work with their families to make this difficult and trying time easier. I have worked hard to earn the trust of parents with colicky babies, and as the first stop on the road to wellness I have gladly accepted this opportunity and challenge to affect change on a grander scale.

Chapter 3

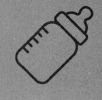

Why Do Babies Cry?

Welcome to the world, little one! The first thing a newborn does is cry. Everyone knows what a crying baby looks like: the baby's face is red; his eyes are closed, mouth is open, and brows are wrinkled; and he may flail his arms and legs. His eyes may not be wet with tears, as babies typically do not have tears until about 1 to 2 months of age. Also, in the first couple of weeks after birth, the crying occurs more for bodily reasons (eg, hunger, hiccups, startles, acid reflux) than psychological or emotional (eg, anger, boredom). But what is the purpose of the cry? It is a distress signal: "I'm uncomfortable!" It is a form of communication: "I'm hungry! I'm hurt!" Your crying baby tells you that he is uncomfortable and upset and has reached his limit. It is rare for a baby to never cry; if your baby never cries, discuss this with your pediatrician. According to pediatrician T. Berry Brazelton, MD, there is a "normal curve of crying": from birth to 8 weeks of age, the average amount of crying is 2.4 hours per day; from 8 to 12 weeks, babies cry an average of less than 1 hour per day. There is also a "witching hour" every day, typically in the late afternoon or early evening, when most babies cry and nothing seems to help—no strategy you use stops the crying. (See Chapter 5 for more information about sensory processing.) Developmentally, crying peaks at 6 weeks of age and gradually decreases at around 4 months of age. Of course, these are just averages, and there is much variation from baby to baby. Fussy babies, especially, cry much more than the typical baby—at least 3 hours per day.

With technology today you can track just about anything about your baby—feeding and sleeping habits, elimination output, developmental milestones, growth, medicine intake—and even share memorable moments and photos privately. There was a recent study in Canada about providing a list of quality parenting apps to parents. The initial search came up with 4,300 free apps for new parents! That is very overwhelming; which one do you choose, how many do you use, and what do you do with all that data about your baby? This can be very anxiety provoking; some might consider it another stressful responsibility you are encouraged to do as a new parent. The study divided the apps into 5 categories according to their primary purpose: tracking, informational, sleeping aid, photo sharing, and miscellaneous. The study used a MARS (Mobile App Rating Scale) tool to evaluate each app and included 4 subscales: engagement, functionality, aesthetics, and information (the subscale we believe is most critical; this is the quality, quantity, and credibility of information on the app). One goal of this study was to find an avenue to assist parents in identifying risks and benefits associated with a particular app. Another was to encourage health care professionals to support digital literacy among parents of babies they treat and have quality information about apps that they recommend.

There are good things about these apps, and the reality is that you as a new parent may end up using 1 or more of these apps. They can keep your life organized, provide a positive way to share information with your primary care physician, and are a good support to new parents in terms of convenience and immediate assistance. Be cognizant of some disadvantages as well. These apps can keep you tethered to your phone, provide inaccurate or unreliable information, and take away from watching your baby and developing your own parenting instincts. Bottom line: choose cautiously. Look for privacy policies, check the source of the information, and appreciate the process of learning about your own baby.

When parents bring their baby to our clinic, we have them complete a Behavior Diary (Figure 3.1) for 3 to 5 days to find out exactly how often their baby cries, how long the crying lasts, and when the crying happens the most. We then analyze this information to gain a greater understanding about their baby's crying. This is different than the baby apps many parents are completing on a daily basis. With this behavior diary, we are looking at just 5 behaviors (sleeping, crying, fussing, eating, and awake time) for only 3 to 5 days to see if there is any pattern that we could adjust.

The Behavior Diary tells us several things. First, it tells us how much the baby cries as well as how much the baby fusses. If the baby cries more than 3 hours a day for 3 days, this is above average and typically would fall under the colic diagnosis. Still, not all babies who are fussy are diagnosed with colic; they may just be considered as babies with excessive fussiness. Second, the diary identifies if there is a pattern to the crying; for example, crying after feedings, increased crying during the early evening, or a longer period of crying that is

SAMPLE BEHAVIOR DIARY

DAY 1 4/20/21

AM

Midnight	12:15 AM	12:30 AM	12:45 AM	1:00 AM	1:15 AM	1:30 AM	1:45 AM	2:00 AM	2:15 AM	2:30 AM	2:45 AM	3:00 AM	3:15 AM	3:30 AM	3:45 AM	4:00 AM	4:15 AM	4:30 AM	4:45 AM	5:00 AM	5:15 AM	5:30 AM	5:45 AM
S	S	S	S	S	S	S	S	S	S	S	S	E	E	S	S	S	S	S	S	S	E	A	A

6:00 AM	6:15 AM	6:30 AM	6:45 AM	7:00 AM	7:15 AM	7:30 AM	7:45 AM	8:00 AM	8:15 AM	8:30 AM	8:45 AM	9:00 AM	9:15 AM	9:30 AM	9:45 AM	10:00 AM	10:15 AM	10:30 AM	10:45 AM	11:00 AM	11:15 AM	11:30 AM	11:45 AM
A	F	F	C	S	S	S	S	S	E	E	A	A	F	F	F	C	C	S	F	F	E	E	E

PM

Noon	12:15 PM	12:30 PM	12:45 PM	1:00 PM	1:15 PM	1:30 PM	1:45 PM	2:00 PM	2:15 PM	2:30 PM	2:45 PM	3:00 PM	3:15 PM	3:30 PM	3:45 PM	4:00 PM	4:15 PM	4:30 PM	4:45 PM	5:00 PM	5:15 PM	5:30 PM	5:45 PM
S	S	S	S	S	S	S	S	A	A	E	E	A	A	A	F	F	C	C	C	E	E	F	F

6:00 PM	6:15 PM	6:30 PM	6:45 PM	7:00 PM	7:15 PM	7:30 PM	7:45 PM	8:00 PM	8:15 PM	8:30 PM	8:45 PM	9:00 PM	9:15 PM	9:30 PM	9:45 PM	10:00 PM	10:15 PM	10:30 PM	10:45 PM	11:00 PM	11:15 PM	11:30 PM	11:45 PM
F	S	S	S	S	S	S	S	S	E	E	E	E	E	S	S	S	S	S	S	S	S	S	S

Baby Behavior

S = *sleeping*   E = *eating*   C = *crying*   F = *fussing*   A = *awake (content)*

Figure 3.1. Behavior Diary

at a consistent time every day. It also gives us an idea of your baby's patterns for sleep and feeding. Are his sleep and feeding schedules inconsistent, or are they somewhat predictable across the days? Are the feedings equally spaced throughout the day? Does your baby have long periods of awake time, which leads to overtiredness? Finally, it helps to get some perspective on your baby's crying; is it truly abnormal, or does it just feel that way? Take a look at the Sample Behavior Diary (Figure 3.1) in this chapter of a 2-month-old fussy baby girl. As you can see when we look at 1 day, or 24 hours, the baby sleeps fairly well at night and has a fussy time in the afternoon, but what is apparent is that the baby does not sleep much during the day. She wakes at 8:00 am and the first nap is not until noon. As discussed in other chapters in this book, we need to look at how long babies are awake (Chapter 9) and learn to read their cues (Chapter 4). This baby may be tired during the fussy late morning time, she may be giving subtle cues that the parent is missing, or the parent may be trying to get her to sleep during that time and the baby is fighting sleep. It is also possible that the parent may have missed the window for sleep and, because the baby is overtired, she is much harder to get to sleep, leading to fussing and crying.

In Resources, we have provided you a blank Behavior Diary to use with your own baby. Complete this Behavior Diary for your baby for 3 to 5 days. The behaviors to highlight are sleeping, eating, crying, fussing, and being awake. Place a letter in each box (eg, sleeping = S; eating = E). (Refer to the crying/fussing chart that follows to see the difference between crying and fussing.) The diary is divided into 15-minute increments. Look at each 15-minute increment and list the behavior you see for most of those 15 minutes (eg, if your baby eats for 10 minutes, write an E). So, if your baby sleeps from midnight to 3:00 am, write an S in each 15-minute increment box over that period. If he wakes up and eats for 5 to 15 minutes, write an E in the corresponding box. If he goes back to sleep, continue to write an S in the boxes until he wakes up. Keep the diary with you so you can write down the behaviors you see; it is too hard to remember the behaviors at the end of the day. Once you have completed the diary, use 5 different markers (1 color for each behavior) and color-code the behaviors that you see. This gives you a good visual view to help you analyze your baby's behavior. Sometimes there is a clear pattern that you have not been aware of. It's worth a try to help you better understand your baby.

There can be a spectrum of behaviors from fussing to full-blown crying. Fussing is often a warning sign that crying is about to happen. But sometimes a baby only fusses a lot, which does not always lead to crying. The following chart shows some of the differences between crying and fussing.

Crying	Fussing
High-pitched sound	Lower pitched sound
Open mouth posture	No open mouth
Body is tense.	Body is squirmy and active.
Brow is wrinkled.	Eyebrows angle up.
"Cry face"	"Pouting face"

Often, when we hear a baby cry, our first instinct is to try and stop the crying. What is even *more* important is to see if we can figure out *why* the baby is crying. Then maybe we can address that need! If we pay attention to the cries—really look and listen—and read other cues that lead up to crying, we may learn what those cries mean. There are many types of crying, and some babies have clear cries that indicate what they need. Fussy babies do not always have clear cries. Some professionals think that babies only have 2 cries, pain and everything else. We tend to think babies have more than 2 cries with all of them trying to communicate something. Table 3.1 provides some examples of different types of cries and some possible solutions; see if you recognize the different cries in your baby. Remember, not all of these cries are seen in every baby, so really watch your baby and learn about his cries!

You can see and hear the variations in *how* a baby cries: how loud it is, how high-pitched it is, how long it lasts, and what makes it stop. There may also be clues in what happened right before the crying started and how quickly the baby escalated to crying. Was he fussing a little, then getting louder and louder, and then reaching full crying? In comparison, fussy, colicky, and high-need babies often do *not* have clear cries, and parents may have a hard time figuring out what is wrong and what the baby needs. The other thing to remember is that you are most likely exhausted because you have not been sleeping well. Think of when you are at work on a day you have not slept well; you are less than your optimal self. So, this exhaustion affects your ability to be alert and sensitive to the cries of your baby.

Explanations of crying that are specific to a fussy or colicky baby include

- **Intense crying.** In the case of intense, hysterical crying, the first course of treatment is to call your pediatrician to rule out medical reasons.

- **Nonspecific-related crying.** Treatment for persistent crying (ie, not necessarily screaming, so not as distinct as intense crying) is usually support and behavioral interventions.
- **Feeding-related crying.** This type of crying is seen during feeding with screaming, turning away frequently, or feeding well for a short time and then pulling away and crying. Treatment includes referral to a lactation consultant and/or a speech-language pathologist specializing in infant feeding.

Table 3.1. What Are the Different Types of Cries?

Type of Cry	Differentiating Characteristics	Solutions to Try
Hunger	This cry is a short, continuous burst; insistent and medium pitched, it is often steady and rhythmic, like "waa, waa, waa." The rooting response is often seen when hungry, prior to the start of crying. It often escalates when you don't start the feeding. If you feed your baby and she stops and starts to look around, it might not have been a hunger cry.	The obvious solution is to try and feed your baby![a] If you are breastfeeding, offer the breast. If you are bottle-feeding and the bottle isn't ready to go, give your baby a pacifier.[b] She will suck briefly and realize this is *not* food, and this may escalate the crying—she will *not* be happy! But that communicates that yes, she really *is* hungry, and confirms this is her hunger cry. It's not always easy to prepare the bottle ahead of time and to be ready when your baby is hungry. If you are bottle-feeding you can have your partner help prepare the bottle while you are trying to calm your baby and getting her ready to eat.
Fatigue	A fatigue cry is usually a soft, rhythmical cry or a whimpering that builds up quickly to the peak of a loud, distressed cry. If you don't "catch" it she sometimes gets to the "point of no return," and your baby is then overtired.	Try to get her to sleep if sleep is due. Look at awake times (see Chapter 9), see when the last time she slept was, and determine if she is reaching that overtired point.

Boredom	This is a "fake" cry, with some whimpering in bursts, but it is not constant. These are more noises of annoyance than a true cry. He may stop when he can entertain himself. He may find his hand and start playing but then go back to whimpering. In essence, he wants your attention!	Try talking to him! The sound of your voice gives him what he needs: your attention! You can also try to change his position or the environment, such as changing the room he is in or the toys around him. If he still fusses, pick him up, as the crying will usually stop when he truly is bored. However, once he is calm, place him back down but in a different position.
Discomfort	This cry is typically less piercing with bursts of crying and is typically not as "disturbing" as a pain cry. It sounds like a boredom cry but doesn't stop when you pick him up.	Sometimes your baby is too hot or too cold, so change the layers of clothing. He may need a diaper change. He also may have gas or needs to have a bowel movement. If so, a tummy massage may help. The tummy position is a great position to use to provide firm pressure on the tummy if he is gassy or needs to have a bowel movement. Sometimes babies are just uncomfortable because they ate too much and may need to burp or just be held upright. You can try to burp him, but if a burp doesn't come up that is OK; don't keep patting him.
Pain	A pain cry is a short, sharp scream or a loud, piercing wail. It is an unmistakable shrill sound that often comes out of nowhere. It is often high pitched; sometimes, the breath is held, which is then followed by another scream.	This solution is difficult. If the pain is temporary (eg, a shot), you usually can hold and comfort your baby until he recovers and calms. If the pain lingers (eg, ear infection), the holding and comforting doesn't always work. Then you need to call your pediatrician and have the pediatrician rule out any medical issues.

[a] If you are having difficulty feeding your baby, review Chapter 10 on feeding challenges.
[b] Some breastfeeding experts suggest that use of a pacifier is best introduced when maternal milk supply and breastfeeding is established in the first 3 weeks. In times of fussiness not related to hunger, however, the pacifier may be useful in avoiding unnecessary supplementation.

Say Less, Listen More

It is OK to feel discouraged at times. Getting to know your baby takes time, and learning what your baby's cues mean also takes time. Take time to watch and listen to your baby. Zack Boukydis, PhD, a developmental-clinical psychologist whose career was devoted to working with mothers, families, and babies, stated: "Say less; watch and listen more." This is what helps you understand your baby. So, take the time to really listen and watch your baby. You will hear this throughout the book because it is very important to listen and watch your baby. Don't rely on an app that tells you about your baby's cries; rely on your observations. (See Chapter 4 for more information on reading your baby's cues.)

Child Abuse Is Preventable

Crying elicits many emotions in parents. When you understand your baby and can help him, you feel good. But when you don't know how to help your baby, you may start to feel helpless or inadequate or insecure about your competence as a parent. This can lead to frustration, anger, or even injuring the baby out of desperation. We want to prevent this; shaking a baby should *never* happen, as it can cause irreversible damage to the baby's brain and even death.

Shaken baby syndrome, a form of abusive head trauma, is preventable. If you feel overwhelmed, place your baby down in a safe place, such as a crib or bassinet, and walk away or sit with your baby. (I remember doing that with my baby. I simply sat there and cried along with him!) Make sure you find ways to relieve your stress. Have a plan when you find yourself frustrated that includes who you will call and what will you say. You can call your primary care physician or the registered nurse at the physician's office. You can try to pass your baby off to your partner for a turn and go for a walk or take a shower. You can also call a friend or family member for some needed emotional support. Check in with your pediatrician to make sure you baby does not have a medical problem, or especially if you think your baby may have been injured.

Self-soothing Techniques

Along with learning about your baby's cries, it is important to learn to recognize and support your baby's efforts to self-soothe. Babies need their parents to help soothe them until they are able to do it themselves. This is called *dependent soothing* and is a normal part of newborn care. This includes nursing your baby, holding her, swaddling her, skin-to-skin contact, or rocking her until she calms down. *Self-soothing* or *self-calming* is the ability for a baby to calm down on her own, without help from parents, by sucking her thumb, bringing her hands together, or grabbing onto her blanket (see list at the end of this section). Babies are unable to calm themselves very well before 9 weeks of age, and the ability to self-soothe varies widely from baby to baby. In the early weeks, your baby can self-soothe when mildly upset, usually by sucking her finger, thumb, or fist. However, she cannot always sustain sucking because it is not well coordinated yet. Her hand moves away from her mouth, or she can't get the rhythm going on her thumb. This adds to her frustration and sometimes leads to startling, and her hand jumps farther away from her mouth. Some babies self-calm very easily by just sucking their thumbs, while other babies do not self-calm well and rely on their caregiver to calm them. Some babies may just need a little help to calm down, which is called *assisted calming*. For example, you might put a pacifier in the baby's mouth, change his position by rolling him to his side, assist in getting his thumb to his mouth, or put him in a baby swing, while awake. A baby should *always* be supervised when in a swing due to the risk of positional asphyxia (see "Positional Asphyxia" text box later in this chapter). You can help your baby learn strategies to self-soothe and stop crying, so your baby does not have to depend completely on a parent to be soothed.

Your baby may show attempts at self-soothing at birth and may need help developing those skills. Some attempts can be easy to recognize, while some are not so easy. Certain positions make self-soothing easier; for example, babies will naturally roll to their side into a flexed fetal position in an effort to self-calm. (See more about positioning in Chapter 12.)

Here are some examples of attempts of young babies to self-soothe. Do you see any of these attempts in your baby?

- One or both hands to mouth or face
- Hands clasped together or crossing arms across chest
- Grasps and holds on to parent's finger or blanket
- Crossing legs
- Visually fixing on stimuli in the environment such as a light or colorful object
- Paying attention to voices or faces near to them
- Sucking on finger, thumb, or hand (not hunger)
- Making fists and putting them by ears
- Extending the legs or bracing against parent or crib
- Fetal position ("curled up" posture), sometimes against crib wall
- Rolling from lying on the back to on the side
- Bringing feet together
- Touching a foot to a leg and holding
- Stroking face or body
- Averting gaze and either maintaining an awake state or shifting to a drowsy state

Positional Asphyxia

Positional asphyxia occurs most frequently in babies when they don't receive enough oxygen to breathe due to the position of their body. This can happen in car seats, bouncers, carrying devices, slings, strollers, and swings. It can occur when babies do not have strong head control and their chin compresses into their chest. Positional asphyxia also occurs when babies' mouth and nose are blocked or when their chest cannot fully expand for a breath. This happens when buckles are too loose or are partially buckled and babies slide down in the device. It is imperative to ensure that babies are *always* buckled into devices correctly. With baby wearing, make sure you can always see their face, which must not be covered by fabric. Never leave babies unsupervised in any of these devices.

Positional asphyxia most frequently occurs when babies sleep in these devices. According to the American Academy of Pediatrics, babies should *not* be placed in these devices to sleep. (See Chapter 9 for more information on safe sleeping practices.)

The Importance of Self-soothing

To be able to self-soothe is an important milestone in development and an important life skill. The term *self-soothing* can sometimes be interpreted as a parent making a baby cry it out or ignoring your baby's cries. This is absolutely not true. Allowing babies to learn these calming strategies provides them with the ability to be more autonomous and independent and not to be dependent on their parents to calm them. It is definitely a learning curve! Self-soothing is talked about a lot in reference to sleep, but it is also important as your baby grows to be able to self-soothe or cope when she doesn't get a toy, when you leave the room, etc. If we can lead by example and teach good coping skills from the beginning, we will have a happy, well-adjusted child. When you can teach your baby to self-soothe it helps you as a parent to trust your intuitive competency.

Did You Know?

Did you know the neonatal intensive care unit (NICU) uses facilitated tucking? The baby is rolled to the side and his arms and legs are brought toward the torso, like a fetal position. The NICU staff use this during daily care and during painful procedures such as heel sticks. It is a naturally calming and organizing position, and research has shown that neonates have decreased reaction to pain when held in this position.

Progression of Soothing Techniques

I (Patti) lead a progression of techniques for parents when they are trying to teach their baby to soothe. This is a progression you can use to help babies with colic, but it also can help typical babies who are simply having a fussy time on a certain day. If your baby is extremely irritable, he may be hungry (and then you need to feed him) or very tired (and then you need to try to help him sleep). If you think your baby is in pain, you need to address that. If all of these are ruled out and your baby is fed, changed, and well rested but fussy, then you can try this progression of self-soothing. Too often, when your baby is crying (which may seem like all the time!), you may have the instinct to immediately pick him up. Instead, next time try this progression to help him calm. This progression helps to slow down and really learn about your baby and what he needs. Make sure to wait between each effort to see how he responds. Try each technique slowly, and pause to see how your baby responds; you will both learn what helps and what doesn't. The order of the progression is important because you are doing less at the beginning by just using your voice and more at the end when you are holding and possibly feeding your baby. The goal is for your baby to calm with less intervention from you and for you to move away from holding your baby all day, something that happens frequently with fussy babies.

The CALM Baby Method progression

- Look at your baby, letting her see your eyes.
- Look at her and talk to her.
- Put a hand on her belly or chest.
- Hold her arms together in toward the body or curl her legs up toward her belly.
- Change her position by rolling her onto her side.
- Pick up your baby and hold her in your arms or at your shoulder (but don't move yet!).
- Hold and rock your baby.
- Swaddle your baby and rock her.
- Place a pacifier in her mouth (or assist her to get her hand or thumb to her mouth to suck). You can also try this earlier in the progression if your baby likes pacifiers.
- Feed her if you think this will help.

Other strategies you can incorporate include massaging her back while you are holding her, singing to her, walking with her, and using white noise. When babies are extremely fussy, we tend to try many things to help them calm. But sometimes this means we are adding more stimulation to an already overwhelmed sensory system, and this can be counterproductive. You may hold her, walk around, change positions, pat, sing, pass her on to your partner, etc, and this is too much input. Some parents I have worked with choose an intense strategy, such as sitting on a gymnastics ball and bouncing; however, this is risky, as your baby's head control may not be strong enough to handle this intense movement or you could accidentally fall off the ball with your baby in your arms. When babies are inconsolable,

I advise parents to try 1 strategy (1 or 2 sensory inputs) for about 5 minutes before moving on the next. This may seem like a long time, but it allows your baby to process the sensations and gives her time to settle. A great position to try is the Hanging Out position (see Chapter 12 for more information on postural control). It may take a couple of minutes for her to settle, and sometimes you may hear an escalation in her crying right before she settles into the position. Other things you can try include standing up and holding your baby firmly while she is sucking on a pacifier, shushing or patting her, and swaddling and rocking her—but **do not** attempt all the strategies at once or in too quick succession, or she will get overstimulated! We also talk about decreasing the intensity of the input or the interaction; talk more quietly, move more slowly, use less animation in your face. Try to stick with 1 method for 5 minutes; if it does not help your baby calm, move on to a different strategy and give that 5 minutes. Give each strategy a good try before giving up. Every time your baby cries, try the strategy, and do this for 1 or more days to see if it helps your baby to make a change. If you feel like a certain strategy works some of the time, try that one first. Consistency is key when trying to establish some behaviors. Your baby might not stop fussing immediately, but as you are implementing the strategy each time she cries, she may be getting used to the strategy and may calm more quickly over time. Remember that mom may have a strategy that works for her and dad may have a different strategy that works for him, and this is absolutely fine!

As babies get older, their cries change, and so should your strategies to help them calm. They should become less dependent on you to help them calm. Again, this varies from baby to baby. Sometimes parents find a strategy that works well with their baby, such as doing squats with their baby in their arms, that is much more difficult to do with an older, heavier baby! Parents tend to stay with strategies that once worked and may be reluctant to try something different, fearing that it might not work. Babies can get too big for a baby swing, or a parent bouncing a baby while sitting on a gymnastic ball could be more difficult or even risk a fall as the baby gets heavier. Be open to when it is time to try something different that may be more suitable or safer for your baby as she grows.

If you and your baby are still frustrated, there are more resources (see Resources) that can help you. Consider getting help from a pediatric occupational therapist who specializes in treating infants, an infant mental health specialist, or a pediatric developmental psychologist. These professionals can help you understand your baby, help you learn how to read his cues, and help you promote self-regulation. You are the consumer, so interview these professionals to make sure they have the professional experience you are looking for to have the best chance of success.

> "It was very helpful to learn that fussy babies don't always have clear meaning behind their cries. I felt as if I didn't understand my baby. I am learning her hunger cry the best, but her other cries are still hard to distinguish. But by watching her I am learning what those cries mean, knowing it will take time."
>
> Mother of a 2-month-old fussy baby

Chapter 4

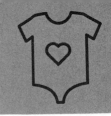

Reading Cues: What Is Your Baby Saying?

Managing your baby's crying, sleeping, and feeding can be overwhelming in the first couple months after birth. If you can understand your baby better, your stress level decreases and your competence and confidence about your parenting skills increase because you are learning *how* to communicate with your baby. Babies have a special language all their own. As discussed in Chapter 3, crying is their *primary* way to communicate. Babies also have other subtle ways of communicating too: with body movement and postures, facial gestures or expressions, and other sounds such as whimpering and cooing.

Reading Baby's Cues

Kevin Nugent, PhD, of the Brazelton Institute and well-known expert on newborn behavior and parent-child relationships wrote a beautifully illustrated book about reading baby's cues. *Your Baby Is Speaking to You: A Visual Guide to the Amazing Behaviors of Your Newborn* and *Growing Baby* includes some of the most gorgeous baby pictures I have ever seen and teaches you about the amazing ways your baby communicates, from subtle cues to clear cues through body language, social language, and expressions.

Infant development specialists have labeled these nonverbal forms of communication as *cues*. All babies are wired to connect with you and learn from you, and they communicate this with these cues. Cues are signals or messages that your baby is trying to tell you and are typically identified in

2 distinct ways: *engaging* (or stable) and *disengaging* (or stress) cues. Engaging cues communicate that your baby is comfortable and ready for interaction. These are fun and easy to read! Disengaging cues mean that your baby is not comfortable with what is going on and needs to take a break. All babies show both types, but, unfortunately, fussy babies show disengaging cues more often than not. In the early days and weeks after birth, trying to figure out what your baby is saying seems like a guessing game. *What is he trying to tell me?* You are sleep deprived and exhausted, which it makes it even more difficult to have patience to learn about your baby's cues. Allow yourself to focus on both of you getting to know each other during those beginning days and weeks.

Did You Know?

There is a program in Germany at the MenschensKind clinic that works with fussy babies and their parents using guided parent-infant training sessions within a developmental-psychological context. The idea for this program came out of the understanding that parents with fussy babies have no idea why the babies are fussing and crying so much and, therefore, resort to misguided strategies to help calm their babies, such as excessive driving in a car, pushing in a stroller, constant feeding, or bouncing on a large therapy ball. The goal of this program is to help parents read or decode their baby's language. They have parents and their baby stay for a 2-hour "baby reading hour" and encourage parents to bring their baby at a fussy time. The therapists resist taking the baby to calm and work with the family to develop some successful strategies.

Factors That Affect Delivery of Cues

Engaging or disengaging cues are affected by 4 factors that allow your baby to be either calm and organized or fussy and irritable. These factors include

- **The environment.** We will learn about the importance of the environment in Chapter 5 with your baby's sensory world. Loud sounds, bright lights, changes in temperature, and handling your baby all have the potential to disorganize your baby, followed by the cues listed later in this chapter in Table 4.1.

- **The baby's arousal level.** This determines how alert or sleepy he is. (See Table 4.1.) Cues correspond with certain arousal levels; the "I want to play, socialize, and learn!" cue always happens in the quiet alert state; conversely, the "I need a break! I need my space!" cue always happens in the active alert state.
- **Motor function.** This refers to a baby's postural control and movement patterns, as we will learn in Chapter 12. Your baby's motor stability tells you whether he is coping with the environment. (See Table 4.1.)
- **Physiological state.** This describes your baby's heart and breathing rates. Your baby's skin tone also tells you how comfortable he is.

If you have a hard time reading and understanding your baby's cues (which is very characteristic of fussy babies), it is difficult to respond to them in an effective way. When you start to understand what your baby is trying to tell you, you can start to respond to those cues with the correct answer. The joy that comes with parenting a baby who is content, easy to read, and easy to soothe is often lost with fussy babies.

Thankfully, research on infant development has led to the understanding that babies do communicate; they are social beings who use nonverbal body language to communicate their wants and needs. The key with learning is watching them intently. You are the one who can learn and get to know your baby the best by watching her. (See Chapter 3 for soothing strategies and Chapter 5 for the effects of sensory input.) Every one of your baby's signals may be trying to tell you something. Cues tell us about her wants and needs, her likes and dislikes. They can tell you if she needs food, comfort, stimulation, or simply a little quiet time. This is why it is so important to try to learn your baby's cues: it makes everyone's life easier. As you learn your baby's unique cues, share each bit of new understanding with other caregivers and family members. As you become an expert on understanding your baby's cues, your baby will also become clearer in sending her messages. By getting a reliable response from her parent, she is learning, "When I do *this*, Mom and Dad will do *that*." You are learning about each other!

Recognizing Your Baby's Cues

Every baby's cues are different. Some babies give very clear, obvious cues. These babies are much easier to care for. Fussy or high-need babies either don't give a lot of cues or give such subtle cues that we often miss them, so they are harder to interpret. They also may give cues that mean more than one thing. At one time, sucking on her hand may mean, "I'm hungry"; another time, it may mean, "I'm upset and need to calm down." The best way to learn your baby's cues is to simply and attentively *watch her*. As we previously advised, say less; watch and listen more. Be patient; this takes time! In the early weeks, you are barely getting enough sleep to be alert yourself, so it is hard to be attuned to what your baby is trying to convey. But learning to read her cues is the *best* way to understand your baby. Try to take several minutes at different times of the day and just watch your baby. That means putting down the phone, turning off the TV, shutting down the computer, holding off on the chores, and just watch her while she is feeding, during playtime, when she is being held by your partner, when she is fussy, when she is sleepy, and even when she is asleep. These moments of pure observation may feel like missed opportunities to respond to your baby, but observation is very different than ignoring. Observation is a response, and one that will instinctively lead to a host of new responses that you cultivate as you come to better understand your baby. The more you watch her, the more you will learn.

The Meaning Behind the Cues

Babies have a rich repertoire of behaviors and a lot of cues that all mean different things. Appreciate and learn your baby's uniqueness. Watch your baby's whole body; she could be giving more than 1 cue at a time. Some cues mean different things depending on the time of day. Don't get discouraged; it's a learning process. When you see a cue, observe the behavior and respond to what you think it means: "Oh, you must be tired, hungry, etc." If you don't get it right the first time, try something else!

Table 4.1 is not an all-inclusive list; it is a guide. Your baby may show you cues not on this list or may not show many of these cues. Trust your gut and interpret what you see in your baby! Keep confident that you can learn to read your baby's cues correctly. Sometimes refer to the clock to help you read the cue; for example, identify the last time she ate or how long she has been awake. Don't rely on outside technology, such as an app, that tells you about your baby; let your baby tell you.

Table 4.1 What Is Your Baby Saying?

Here are some examples of babies' needs and the cues they may show. Cues with asterisks (*) may mean different things and are listed more than once. Note that different types of cues may be used to express the same thing!

What Your Baby Is "Saying"	Motor System	Baby Cues
I want to play, socialize, and learn!	Face/ expression	Eye contact—may be wide-eyed or narrow focus
		Bright-eyed look
		Mutual gaze
		Looks at your face*
		Smiling—from a little grin to a dazzling social smile (typically starts around 6–8 weeks)
		"Pre-reaching": eyes wide and bright, eyebrows rise, mouth opens—"reaching with her eyes"
		Mouth opens, jaw drops
	Body/ posture/ movements	Turns toward you
		Raises head toward you
		Reaches toward you, arms activate
		Smooth arm and leg movements with a still body
	Vocalizing	Coos (typically starts around 6–8 weeks)
		Grunts, whimpers, or coughs may mean, "I want your attention."
I'm hungry!	Face/ expression	Moves mouth/lips in sucking motions, lip-smacking, pursing lips, loud "feeding" sounds
		Opens mouth to accept the breast or bottle nipple
		Sucks vigorously on the nipple, either breast or bottle
		Looks at your face*
		Sticks out tongue*
		Sucks on hands,* pacifier, anything placed near baby's mouth
		Increased alertness

continued

Table 4.1 (*continued*)

What Your Baby Is "Saying"	Motor System	Baby Cues
I'm hungry! (*continued*)	Body/posture/movements	Rooting reflex: baby's face turns toward a light touch on the cheek (This response may not mean hunger, so pay attention to when this is happening)
		Nuzzles mother's breast
		Gets excited at the sight of the breast or bottle
		Leans toward or reaches for the bottle
		Moves head restlessly from side to side*
		Increased physical activity
		Arches back*
		Hand/finger to mouth*
		Flexes arms and legs
		Clenches fingers and fists*
	Vocalizing	Rapid breathing as a prelude to crying*
		Fusses*; leads to crying if not fed
I'm full; I've had plenty!	Face/expression	Sucking slowing down, with breaks
		On and off the nipple (bottle or breast); may push it out of mouth
		Stops nursing or taking a bottle
		Smiles—sometimes just a pause for a social smile; pay attention to baby's timing.
		Looks settled and relaxed; may be falling asleep*
		Relaxes jaw; closes lips
		Clamps mouth shut
	Body/posture/movements	Turns head away
		Pushes away
		Arms and legs are stretched out
		Fingers relax and open
		Shows more interest in surroundings
	Vocalizing	Sighs

What Your Baby Is "Saying"	Motor System	Baby Cues
I need some help to settle, calm, get organized!	Face/ expression	"Cry face": wrinkled, puckered, furrowed brow*
		Frowns*
		Tongue thrusts
	Body/ posture/ movements	Fidgets, squirms, strains to change position, arches back*
		Flails; uncoordinated movement*
		Increased body activity in supine position
		Braces hands or feet against crib, stretching leg muscles
		Pushes hand toward you
		Rolls to the side*
		Sucks on hands*
		Sweats on back of head or neck
		Clasping hands
		Hand to mouth, ear*
		Hands behind head*
		Grasps tightly to your shirt
	Vocalizing	Fusses/cries
I'm tired!	Face/ expression	Eyes dull, glazed, unfocused; drowsy, heavy eyes, staring in space OR
		Eyes wide open,* unblinking
		Yawns*
		Looks away from people and toys (gaze aversion)*
		Eyes slowly close and spring open again and again
		Face and jaw limp, relaxed
		Frowns*
		Covers face with blanket
		Moves head side to side*

continued

Table 4.1 (*continued*)

What Your Baby Is "Saying"	Motor System	Baby Cues
I'm tired! (*continued*)	Body/ posture/ movements	Sucks on hands*
		Lull in body activity, being still
		Nods head when held upright or while on tummy
		Arches body*
		Tightly clenches fists*
		Flails; uncoordinated movement*
		Jerky arms and legs
		Not settling in your arms
		Rubs nose or eyes
		Puts arms or hands in front of face
		Tugs at ear or hair
		Hand by ear*
		Pulls up knees
		Hiccups*
	Vocalizing	Quiets down in general; less "talkative"
		Whines to cries to screams if no ability or attempts to help fall asleep
I need a break! I need my space!	Face/ expression	Looks away from people and toys (gaze aversion)*
		Gaze locking (eyes locked on 1 stimulus)
		Eyes too wide*
		Eyes shut but not sleepy; may be fretful
		Nostril flares
		Changes in facial color
		Raises eyebrows
		Frowns, grimaces*
		Head fully turns away
		Wrinkles forehead*
		Yawns*

What Your Baby Is "Saying"	Motor System	Baby Cues
I need a break! I need my space! (*continued*)	Body/ posture/ movements	Arches*
		Pulls away
		Jerky, fractious movements
		Kicks, moving body
		Rolls to side in tucked position*
		Salutes/halt hand
		Finger splaying
		Hands by ear*
		Hand to mouth*
		Hand behind head*
		Sucks on hands vigorously*
		Hiccups*
		Fencing reflex: baby turns head to 1 side and stretches that arm out with the other arm bent up. The position gives some stability and control, helping baby to "self-organize"
		Becomes upset with noise: shushing, singing, talking
		Sometimes shuts down or falls asleep*
	Vocalizing	Fusses*
		Cries*
		Screeches

Can You Misread a Cue?

Being able to read your baby's cues accurately is a learning process! Don't feel guilty if you misread a cue! It is easy to misinterpret your baby's cues, especially with a fussy baby; remember, babies don't always give clear cues. If you read the cue of sucking on her hands to mean, "I'm hungry," when the cue or her need was, "I need some help to calm down and get organized," you may feed her too soon; she might start to suck and do a short feeding.

Another misreading may be to think because she is sucking on her hands, she must be teething. Babies suck on their hands to calm but also to play and explore their body. If you think it is teething, you may inadvertently give her medicine for teething pain, when it is not really needed. This is why it is very helpful to watch *all* her motor systems when you are reading a cue. If a baby is sucking or mouthing on her hands and she has a calm body and is not fussing, it probably means she's simply playing.

An easily misread cue can be when your baby turns away. Sometimes this is interpreted to mean that she's bored or not interested in you, but it may mean she's a little overwhelmed and needs a break. Often, I have had parents interpret this as, "My baby doesn't like me," which is not true. She is simply communicating to you that she needs a break. As we have said before, don't rely on a baby app to teach you about your baby when you are the one who can watch her and learn.

You Know Your Baby Best

Learning to read your baby's cues takes time and practice. Reading your baby's cues helps you correctly understand her thresholds for stimulation and helps you to connect with her. Sometimes babies give several cues at one time, and sometimes there will be a mix of engaging (stable) and subtle cues and disengaging (stress) cues. This, of course, makes it even harder to know what they are trying to say. Again, keep watching your baby and learning how these cues look. When I (Patti) am working with families and we are trying to identify a baby's cues, instead of labeling the cues as I see them to the parent, I ask the parent some open-ended questions, such as, "What do you think he is telling us?"; "What do you think that sign means?"; and "What do you think is going on with him?" Then we work together to try and figure it out. These are questions you can ask yourself when you are observing your baby. You can read your baby best when you are rested, calm, and flexible. So don't forget to take care of yourself so you can be there for your baby. Sometimes you will guess wrong, and that's OK! Learn from it and try something different next time. Certainly, consider helpful advice from friends and family, but don't be afraid to go with your gut. You are with your baby the most and see her at all times of the day, and you know your baby best!

> "Once I started reading my baby's cues, I felt like I finally understood what my baby was feeling. It made me feel so much better about my parenting instincts."
>
> Mother of a 5-week-old fussy baby

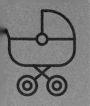
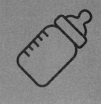

Chapter 5

Your Baby's Sensory World

Babies deal with many new sensations once they are born; they see, hear, smell, taste, and feel/touch. They use their senses to recognize people, objects, and events. At birth, babies' sensory systems are not fully developed. These perceptions are fine-tuned by their life experiences, such as being held and carried, hearing different sounds, touching various toys, and participating in a daily routine such as bathing, diaper changes, and feedings. Sensory input strongly affects the state a baby is in and how he moves through the levels you will learn about in Chapter 6.

Did You Know?

In the uterus, your baby had the cozy protective space of the womb. He received sensory input like the sound of your heartbeat and muffled external sound, being suspended in the amniotic fluid, and movement sensations as you moved around, as well as touch when you would rub your belly or when his thumb found his own mouth or brushed by his body as you moved. Toward the end of pregnancy, he was tightly confined in your uterus, getting deep touch pressure throughout his body.

To fully understand how sensory input affects your baby's levels of arousal, it helps to understand the different sensory systems. The *external* senses are touch, vision, hearing, smell, and taste. There are also 3 other *internal* sensory systems that are not as well known: the movement (*vestibular*) sense, the body position (*proprioceptive*) sense, and the sensations from our internal organs (*interoception*).

External Senses

External senses are the 5 senses that are commonly known. They are the senses that recognize and process sensory input from the environment or the outside world.

Touch

Touch is a fundamental means of interaction between parents and babies. Many studies show the positive effects of touch with babies, including affecting the babies' arousal levels and enhancing the parent-baby relationship. There is comforting touch, such as being cuddled, stroked, massaged, or patted. There is not so comforting touches (pain), such as immunizations. Babies can also recognize cold and hot temperatures. Think of cold air on a warm bottom during a diaper change or going from a warm bath to cold air!

Vision

This sense is the least developed at birth. Babies do see light, as well as contrasts, shapes, and patterns. Research shows that babies prefer looking at faces versus objects, because they can visually process faces before they can recognize objects. Babies can recognize their mother's or father's face and eventually learn to follow a moving object with their eyes between 1 and 3 months of age. Sometimes babies look away when the object is too stimulating; then they recover and come back to look at it again. Babies learn a lot about their world from this sense.

Hearing

Some sounds may be startling to young babies, such as a dog barking or a loud sneeze. They can also be soothed by sounds, such as the sound of their mother's voice or a soft lullaby. (Babies actually can recognize their mother's voice in utero! A fetus will calm to the sound of mom's voice.) As they age, at around 3 to 4 months after birth, they look in the direction of the sound, turn their head, and smile.

Smell

Babies are very sensitive to smells. They recognize a parent's scent, and it makes them feel secure and comforted. Some aromas are too strong; you may notice that your baby may not breastfeed as well if you are wearing a strongly scented lotion or perfume, which is why lactation consultants recommend to not wear lotions and perfume in your baby's first few weeks after birth.

Taste

The sense of taste is closely linked to the sense of smell throughout life. Developmental researchers found that babies can taste sweet and sour at birth but prefer sweetness, so they are primed for breast milk (also known as human milk) by both smell and taste.

Internal Senses

Internal senses are lesser known. You may be aware of them but probably do not know what they are called. These 3 senses recognize and process sensory input that come from within the body.

Movement (Vestibular) Sense

This is known as the vestibular system. It is located within the inner ear. It provides information about head and eye movements, posture, and balance. Babies are comforted by rocking and bouncing, which is vestibular input. But movement can also be disorganizing (distressing); a baby may flail or startle when she is moved too quickly, such as during diaper changes.

Body Position (Proprioceptive) Sense

This is the proprioceptive system. Babies use this sense to naturally adjust their bodies to fit into the arms of the person holding them. It consists of receptors in the muscles, tendons, and joints that provide the perception of movement and position of the body in space. Whether babies are being massaged or are kicking, moving, or lying on their tummy, they receive proprioceptive input, which helps them learn about their body in space. This, in turn, helps with the attainment of future motor skills. Swaddling babies gives them good input to their proprioceptive system, which is very calming and organizing. (See more on swaddling in Chapter 12.)

Sensations From Internal Organs (Interoception)

Interoception describes what is going on inside babies' bodies. They receive messages from their internal organs that convey sensations of hunger, gas discomfort, the need to have a bowel movement or to urinate, or body temperature. These sensations may make babies feel uncomfortable during the early months, but babies' bodies develop the ability to interpret these internal processes as they grow and develop.

The Effects of Sensory Input

Now that we understand the different sensory systems, we can start to see how all these different sensations can affect babies' behavioral states of arousal. Tables 5.1 and 5.2 list each sensory system and the sensory input that either calms and organizes your baby or stimulates and alerts your baby.

Table 5.1 External Sensations and Stimuli That Influence Arousal Levels

Sensory System	Calming/Organizing	Stimulating/Alerting
Touch	Holding Massage Firm patting Swaddling Cuddling Skin-to-skin contact (also called kangaroo care) Steady/firm touch Bring hands together Touch and hold techniques, as in infant massage Sucking on thumb, hands, or pacifier	Light touch Tickling Unpredictable touch Changes in touch pressure (Light touch is more stimulating; deep touch is more calming) Changes in temperature
Hearing	Quiet sounds Consistent sound (white noise) Familiar sounds Rhythmic sounds	Loud noises Unpredictable sounds Unfamiliar sounds Arrhythmic sounds
Taste and smell	Mother's milk Scent of parent Scent of baby Smell of lavender	Unfamiliar smells Strong smells Too many different smells at once (eg, cooking dinner, strong perfumes)

Table 5.2 Internal Sensations and Stimuli That Influence Arousal Levels

Sensory System	Calming/Organizing	Stimulating/Alerting
Movement (vestibular)	Rocking Swaying Gentle bouncing Wearing your baby, as in a sling Slow baby swings	Moving too quickly Unpredictable movement Changing baby's clothes or diaper Baby swings that move a little faster (not recommended if your baby does not have good head control) Being held in the vertical position with less support at the parent's shoulder
Body position (proprioceptive)	Tummy time Being held in the vertical position with support against parent's shoulder Sustained postures Containment (Cradle feet and hold head steady while on his back [also called giving your baby boundaries]) Baby wearing in slings Providing support at head, neck, and trunk as you hold and move your baby Being confined in baby equipment (giving your baby boundaries) Carrying and positioning your baby (See Chapter 12 for ideas)	Lying on their back (Babies startle and move their arms and legs) Being out of baby equipment so they can move and use their muscles Provide less support at head, neck, and trunk as they are getting stronger Gentle baby yoga activities (See Chapter 12 for ideas)
Sensations from internal organs (interoception)	Feeding your baby Colic routine for gas or constipation Tummy time, which provides deep touch pressure to internal organs	*The following sensations are out of your control but affect the arousal level:* Hunger Constipation Gas Needing to eliminate Reflux

You can see from the tables how many different sensory experiences there are that can be calming, stimulating, organizing, or alerting. Understanding the sensory systems and how sensory input affects your baby, and knowing strategies you can use to change their state of arousal, helps with understanding your baby's arousal levels.

Tolerating Sensory Input

Not all babies tolerate sensory input the same way. Some babies are very cuddly and love being held and rocked, and some are not bothered by sounds or sights in their environment. These babies often fall into a deep sleep, wake content, and feed a little easier than other babies. These babies are considered to have easy temperaments. Fussy or high-need babies are often more sensitive to sensory stimuli than typical babies. They react more when you handle or move them during a clothing or diaper change. Even just switching from mom holding the baby to dad is alerting. They often respond to this movement with a strong Moro reflex. The *Moro reflex,* sometimes called the startle reflex, is a normal response to stimulation of movement or loud sounds by flailing their arms and legs and is accompanied by crying. It is present at birth and decreases in intensity toward 2 months of age. This reflex often persists past 2 months of age with fussy or high-need babies and affects their ability to tolerate sensory input on a daily basis. Because this startle often persists with fussy babies, sometimes they need more external support for a longer period of time. Parents inherently know this and hold these babies a little more to help them stay calm and secure. Holding your baby in that curled-up position (called *flexion*) and helping get his hands to midline helps give him boundaries and is much more organizing for him than when he is lying on his back and startling. (See Chapter 12 for more positioning ideas.) The startle response does not go away completely, although it does lessen in intensity—but even into adulthood, we jump at a loud door slam!

Sensory Threshold

Fussy babies may also be more sensitive to touch, so they may not tolerate massaging them, giving them a bath, or wiping after a diaper change. These babies may even resist being touched and cuddled. Sometimes they may feel rigid or stiff because they arch a lot and don't mold into the parent's arms. Parents often worry that their baby doesn't like them, but this is far from the truth. Some fussy babies are not comfortable with touch and movement experiences; it all depends on what their arousal level is. If they are in active and fussy states, they do not tolerate touch and movement as well. It does not mean they don't like you! Their tolerance to sensory input depends on many things, such as the time of day and their level of arousal. When they first wake from sleep, they are often calmer, rested, more organized, and less sensitive to different sensory inputs (unless they are really hungry!). Late afternoon or early evening is sometimes called the "witching hour," when babies tolerate less input. We talk about this in terms of their *sensory threshold*. We all have a sensory threshold; if you are tired, stressed, or not feeling well, your tolerance to sensory input is lower than usual. When a baby reaches his threshold, his behavioral state changes to fussiness or crying and is often difficult to calm. A baby's sensory threshold is on a continuum; it depends on how much sensory input has happened all day. If it has been a busy day with running errands, a doctor appointment, having visitors, etc, your baby may have met his tolerance for sensory input. Babies' sensory overload can build up silently, so sometimes you aren't really aware of it until all of a sudden, they move into that fussy state. In Chapter 4, we discussed reading babies' cues to know when they have had too much or not enough.

Did You Know?

Babies born preterm are at risk for sensory-based difficulties. If you had a baby early who spent any time in the neonatal intensive care unit (NICU) you are aware of all the medical procedures that were required to save your baby's life. Most NICUs do a great job of minimizing overstimulation, but it still does happen. Once babies are stable enough to go home, parents are sent home with a sensitive little baby who has to adjust to a whole new environment. It is found that preemies do fuss and cry more than typical babies because they are often more sensitive and become overstimulated very easily. The solutions highlighted in this book can be used with preemies; however, you may have to slow down the approach or perhaps engage in 1 strategy at a time. You may also have to be less intense with your interactions with them depending on their tolerance. If you are feeling overwhelmed with your preemie at home reach out to your physician and ask for an assessment with an occupational therapist specializing in working with preterm babies. The earlier we can intervene, the more we can help them.

The CALM Zone

There is a zone of optimal arousal or organization that we call the CALM Zone. This is a period when babies are happy, well rested, usually well fed, and in the quiet alert state. Babies can move in 2 ways from this CALM Zone: they can become more stimulated and move into behavioral disorganization, which means an active or fussy state, or they can be under-aroused and in a sleepy drowsy state. (Fussy babies are not often seen in this drowsy state.) As babies grow older, you want them to be in the quiet alert state for longer periods. (See Chapter 6, Figure 6.1, for more about states of arousal.) With fussy babies, try to challenge them to see if you can keep them in that good, organized, quiet alert state for longer. Often, if a fussy baby is in quiet alert, we walk on eggshells to prevent him from getting back to fussy; however, sometimes you need to add a little more sensory input to alert your baby but not to get him too fussy. You can do this by singing a little or dancing gently with him. If he starts to get too aroused, tone it down.

Learning about your baby's cues will help you understand how to interact with your baby. A classic sign of sensory overload, gaze aversion, can be easy to miss. Gaze aversion is when a baby's eyes look away or past you. It suggests 2 different things: either your baby needs to withdraw from the overly demanding situation, or he needs a short break to recover from the excitement of the interaction and may come back to the interaction after recovering. A technique we use in this situation is called *still face*. If your baby looks away, try to keep your face neutral (ie, no smiling or talking) and see if your baby's eyes come back and look at you; this means he is ready for more interaction.

How much babies have slept strongly affects their ability to tolerate sensory input, and we grown-ups are the same way. A well-rested, calm, and organized baby may tolerate her bath or diaper changes better than when she is tired, so take that into consideration with daily care and scheduling routines. Sometimes that means doing a bath earlier in the day when your baby can tolerate it better. Lastly, how the environment appears at any given moment affects your baby's tolerance to sensory input. If the dog is barking, the television is on loudly, and siblings are loud, she may hit her sensory threshold quickly and move into that fussy state. Remember, some interactions are too intrusive or demanding, and it becomes a challenge to focus. Recognize this, lower the intensity, and remember all the sensory systems. Sometimes, if your baby is fussy with clothes being changed, parents should stop talking, singing, or saying, "You're OK," and just quietly get your baby dressed, calming him once fully clothed. Don't stop and try to calm him in the middle of getting dressed; it won't last. If you are aware of this threshold with your baby, it will help you plan your day accordingly. Once you understand your baby's sensory threshold, inform other caregivers about your baby's sensitivity or tolerance for sensory input. This will make life happier and calmer for your baby and everyone around him.

> "When I learned about my daughter's sensory threshold and how it affected her behavior, something just clicked. That's exactly what's 'wrong' with her—she's overstimulated! It made so much sense to me. I was able to use the tables to help explain my daughter's behavior to my husband, parents, in-laws, and friends. I recently gave birth to my son and already I can see a difference in each of their tolerances for sensory input. It is something I am now 'in tune with' on a daily basis with both of my children. No one benefits when everyone is overstimulated and disorganized."
>
> Mother of a formerly fussy baby

Chapter 6

Your Baby's Arousal Levels

All babies cry, sleep, and have fussy times. These are called *arousal levels* or *states of arousal*. There are many other names in the pediatric literature that all really mean the same thing, including *behavioral states, states of consciousness, states of alertness,* and *states of awareness*. States of arousal were first described by Peter H. Wolff, MD, in 1959. Other researchers, such as T. Berry Brazelton, MD, elaborated and refined the concepts in later years. They determined that there are organized patterns to infant behaviors. They defined 6 specific states of arousal, including 3 awake states, 1 transitional state, and 2 sleep states. Each state has its own characteristic behaviors, which are outlined in Table 6.1. Some theorists call them different names, which are also listed in Table 6.1, but they are basically the same 6 states no matter what you call them.

Talk about arousal levels refers to typical newborns and preemies in the neonatal intensive care unit. Once babies grow older, most developmental parenting books and checklists don't discuss arousal levels anymore. However, these arousal levels or behavioral states continue throughout life. Think of the arousal levels you go through as an adult. Everyone sleeps and cycles through quiet sleep and active sleep states. When we sleep, we are in quiet sleep, move to active sleep, and may change positions and then move back to quiet sleep. We also have that transitional state, or drowsy state. This is seen when you are tired but still watching television, and you start to drift off and your head bobs. We also have quiet alert times such as when reading a book or listening to classical music. And as you are aware, we also have active alert states when we are working out, running errands, or have a busy day at work and are on the go all day.

As you learned in Chapter 5, Tables 5.1 and 5.2, there are sensory strategies, both calming/organizing strategies and stimulating/alerting strategies, that can change your baby's arousal level. As adults we also engage in strategies to change our arousal levels. We chew gum, change our position, get up and move around, bounce or shake our leg while sitting, stretch, or fidget; all are an attempt to alert us more so we can pay attention. On the other hand, there are things we do to calm ourselves down when we are too active or too excited, such as deep breathing, moving to a quieter space, or becoming mesmerized on a visual stimulus such as a fish tank or a fireplace. We also know children or adults who seem to be more on the active side—always going, never slowing down—and, on the flip side, people who are generally more sedentary. These are personality differences, or moods, but they are also differences in arousal levels.

Most babies tend to move through 6 states in somewhat predictable patterns. Parents respond naturally as they perform simple strategies to change their baby's level of arousal. For example, parents rock and pat their babies to calm them, moving them to a quiet alert state, or move them around a little if they start to fall asleep during feeding, again moving them to a quiet alert state or an awake state. These babies have what we call good *state regulation* or well-balanced *state control*. Fussy babies tend to be more unpredictable as they move through each of these states and, therefore, have poor state regulation. The simple strategies that work well with a typical baby, such as holding, rocking, or talking, don't work as well with a fussy baby; a fussy baby may move up or down several levels by this stimulation, or it may be hard to get this baby from an active alert to a quiet alert state. State changes can happen due to internal body processes such as gas, reflux, or external stimuli such as visual stimulation and sounds. As listed in Table 6.1, each state is created by an intricate organization of the baby's body systems and responses to stimuli and the environment. These behaviors are described in terms of body activity, eye movement, facial movements, breathing patterns, and response to internal and external stimuli.

The sleep states are much easier to recognize because they are simple—your baby is sleeping! The awake states are a little more subtle and a little harder to recognize (except the crying state!). The way to learn your baby's states of arousal is to keep listening and observing.

States or levels of arousal may progress in either direction, from calm to stimulating or vice versa, as illustrated in Figure 6.1. This is an important concept to understand because you can recognize what your baby needs to

Table 6.1 States of Arousal

State of Arousal	What You See
Deep sleep or quiet sleep	Your baby is sound asleep during this state. His eyes are closed with no body movement. He is not easily awakened by sound; you can move him and he doesn't wake up. You may see some sucking movements occasionally but no other spontaneous movement of the arms or legs. Deep sleep is very restorative. His breathing is smooth and regular.[a]
Active sleep, light sleep, or rapid eye movement (REM) sleep	In this state, your baby is asleep but may move, twitch, or stretch. You may see some grimacing or half-smiles and some sucking movements. You may see small movements of the eyes under the eyelids (REM). Babies are more sensitive to internal stimuli (eg, hunger, gas) and external stimuli (eg, noises, bright lights) than when they are in deep sleep. Your baby will awaken slightly to sound. But he may easily move back to deep sleep, so don't get him up too soon! Sometimes during this state his breathing is a little more irregular, although still typical.
Drowsy, semi-alert, or semi-dozing	This state is a transition state. Your baby may be moving from drowsy to waking up or from drowsy to going to sleep. You will know which way your baby may go depending on if she is just getting up from sleeping or if she is getting tired and moving toward sleep. She may be yawning, or her eyes may be partially open but not well focused, and they may open and close on and off. She may respond to sensory stimuli, although it may be a little sluggish or delayed. In this state, her breathing is a little more irregular.
Quiet alert or awake alert	In this state, your baby is calm and alert. His eyes are open and bright, and he seems to be paying attention to you or his world without moving his body a lot. This is the state where early learning happens because your baby is alert and receptive but not overwhelmed by his surroundings. This is a pleasurable and positive state for parents to experience with their baby because they are most responsive to them. In this state, your baby's breathing patterns are fairly regular.

continued

Table 6.1 (*continued*)

State of Arousal	What You See
Active alert or fussy	Your baby is more physically active and restless during this state. She is a little fussy or cranky but not yet crying. She just seems unsettled, squirmy, or disorganized (active yet fussy). She is more sensitive to stimuli and her breathing is more irregular. In this state your baby is at risk of becoming overstimulated quickly, and that moves her to the crying state. Try some soothing strategies in this state. If they work, it will bring her back down to quiet alert. If they don't work, she will move to the crying state.
Crying	This is an obvious state: your baby is in full-blown crying mode with a strong loud cry. His body may be moving or startling and seems very disorganized. He may straighten or extend his body. His breathing is more irregular during this state. There are many different types of crying and reasons for crying (see Chapter 3).

[a] This does not mean that we want babies to sleep so deeply they cannot be woken up fairly easily (see "What Is SUID?" box in Chapter 9).

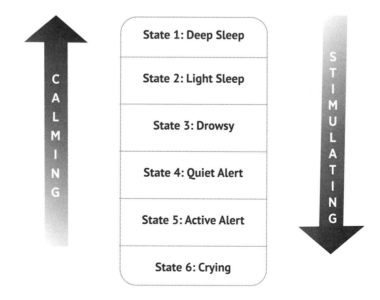

Figure 6.1. The effects of stimulation on state of arousal.

move up or down a level. Babies can move up or down 1 or 2 levels at a time, similar to climbing up and down the rungs of a ladder, depending on the stimuli in their surroundings. They may be in light sleep and slowly awaken through a drowsy state to a quiet alert state simply by being lifted out of their crib. Or they may be crying and move down 2 levels to quiet alert once they start sucking on a pacifier. Much of a baby's behavior throughout the day is organized to bring the baby from a disorganized state (eg, fussy, active alert) to a more organized state (eg, quiet alert, drowsy, sleeping states).

Understanding the Arousal Levels

Understanding your arousal levels helps you understand your baby's arousal levels. It's hard when you are in quiet alert and your baby is in active alert or fussy. Sometimes his level of arousal changes your level of arousal. When you don't understand your baby's arousal levels or when you can't read his cues well, it makes it very difficult to develop successful strategies for changing his arousal if needed, such as getting him to sleep or keeping him awake to feed.

Understanding these levels of arousal is crucial when getting to know your baby and his behaviors in the early days and weeks. Sensory input can influence a baby's level of arousal (see Chapter 5, Tables 5.1 and 5.2). Recognizing these will help you identify strategies you can use to change your baby's state of arousal. In addition, it is beneficial to understand these states to help you strategize about caregiving; for example, if your baby is in the active or fussy state, it might not be the right time for a bath. Some babies move through the different states of arousal fairly predictably; they move through all 6 and do not spend too long in each. A baby can cry but move to quiet alert or drowsy simply by a parent comforting him. As your baby grows older and more mature, he can stay in these states for longer periods; his rate of change between these states depends on his stage of development. That means he can stay in the sleep states (ie, quiet sleep and active sleep) longer, especially at night, which allows you to sleep a little longer. His awake states (ie, quiet alert and active alert) are longer too, allowing for more fun time to play and socialize with you.

Fussy babies tend to spend less time in the sleep states, have shorter sleep phases, fight going to sleep, need more help moving to a sleep state (ie, your help), have more trouble settling to sleep, and wake more frequently.

Did You Know?

Irene Chatoor, MD, a well-known expert in the diagnosis and treatment of children with feeding difficulties, has identified a feeding disorder we sometimes see with fussy babies or babies with colic. It is described as a feeding disorder of state regulation. To feed successfully, babies need to reach and maintain a quiet alert state of arousal. Some babies have difficulties with state regulation during feeding; they are either too irritable and can't calm enough to initiate or continue the feeding, or they are hard to arouse and sleep through a feeding. Fussy babies usually tend toward the former and can't calm for feedings.

This disorder identifies several criteria that are present, including poor and irregular feeding and poor weight gain. A comprehensive assessment of a baby's feeding abilities (by a speech-language pathologist), as well as a thorough assessment of the baby's state management (by an occupational therapist), is indicated to tease out what is going on with these babies. The course of treatment is very different depending on whether a baby has poor feeding skills or poor state management. What is difficult to identify at times is if a baby is very hungry and is irritable and can't settle enough to eat, or if a baby can't coordinate his feeding well enough to get successful intake. Bottom line: if you are having problems feeding your baby find the help you need! (Refer to Chapter 10 for more on feeding.)

Fussy babies also go from a sleep state to crying, whereas typical babies usually wake up to a quiet alert state. Fussy babies are more sensitive to stimulation in their sleep states. They don't habituate (or get used to) negative visual or auditory stimuli when they are sleeping, meaning they can only sleep when it is extremely quiet because any little sound can awaken them. Typical babies aren't always affected by these stimuli and settle right back to sleep, or they may not even pay attention to them if they are in a deep sleep state.

Fussy babies also have difficulty with the awake states, as they frequently are not in that quiet alert or calm state and are more often in the active alert or fussy or crying states. They are often unpredictable, moving restlessly from one state to another in a disorganized way. Their state also changes abruptly and can go from quiet alert to crying without spending any time in the active or fussy state. During fussy babies' awake phases, they may appear hyperalert, hyperexcitable, more irritable, and more susceptible to sensory stimulation. Sometimes, they are hyperreactive to sensory stimuli, which moves them into an active alert state. Sometimes they exhibit pseudo-stability, indicating only a temporary state of calm when moving away from a fussy state. They pay attention to this new stimulus or distraction, but it only lasts a short time and they are back to a fussy state. They also show motor restlessness and are only seldom in a behavioral state of calm attentiveness. They may rarely reach a quiet alert state or a deep sleep state. It may depend on the time of day, how busy the day has been, and the external stimuli around them.

Fussy babies may spend much more time in crying and active alert states and not as much time in quiet alert because they do not regulate their arousal levels well. It is important to understand that one big accomplishment for babies in early infancy is to be able to reach that quiet alert state and maintain this state on their own or with only a little help from parents. This is crucial for optimal brain growth and development. Sometimes parents of fussy babies can be so thrilled that their baby was able to reach this quiet state that they leave their baby alone because they don't want to set them off again for fear of "rocking the boat." However, quiet alert is the best state for early learning, so continue to talk, play, and interact with your baby during this time; watch how strong your input is and the effect it has on your baby!

Did You Know?

The neonatal intensive care unit (NICU) staff uses states of arousals throughout the day as a measurement to understand what arousal level the baby is in at different times throughout the day. The goal of the NICU is to keep a baby in state 1 (deep sleep) or state 4 (quiet alert). Both states are important to achieve to allow a baby to avoid exhaustion, preserve energy, enhance physiological stability, eat well during that quiet alert state, and take time to recover in that deep sleep state. The staff do this by keeping the environment quiet. Some NICUs have a stoplight to alert staff and families if the environment is getting too loud—red light on! Another strategy they use to respect the baby's arousal level is to cluster a baby's care (eg, bath time, measurement of vitals, medical procedures) so a baby has time to recover and is not interrupted several times during the day. Lastly, nurses swaddle babies frequently to help them maintain these positive states of arousal.

Did You Know?

There is a curriculum-based program for preschool and school-aged children called the Zones of Regulation. Designed by an occupational therapist, it was created to help children to identify their feelings and levels of alertness and to learn strategies to change their arousal level for optimal functioning in the classroom or at home. Babies don't have the ability to identify their own arousal levels, but, luckily, parents can identify them in their babies and use strategies to help their baby get to the best state of arousal for the task at hand.

Many of you may have observed these behaviors in your baby, but naming and identifying these arousal levels helps you understand them better and adjust as needed. You can recognize these levels and plan accordingly. If your baby is in an active alert or fussy state, now might not be the time to run to the grocery store, which would add more input to an already over-stimulated nervous system. This is when you may need to recruit some help and not feel like you have to do this on your own. Understanding your baby's states of arousal makes the daily interactions of caring for him a little easier.

> "Understanding that my baby has several levels of arousal helped me to understand her more. Before, I tended to look at her as having 2 states: crying and sleeping! Understanding these levels helped me to plan my day better."
>
> Mother of a 3-month-old fussy baby

Chapter 7

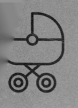

Attachment and the Parent-Baby Relationship

Like all new parents, your first moments of being able to see and hold your new baby are ones that you cherish and fondly recall. An immediate, instinctual bond was formed, and your life was forever changed. A newborn is completely dependent on caregivers for physical and emotional growth. Early experiences with your baby have a great effect on development, and they also form the building blocks for future relationships. When the foundation is strong, babies expect to feel safe and that their needs will be met. This sense of security allows your baby to safely explore her world. As a parent, you also gain confidence and trust when you are able to anticipate your baby's needs and provide loving and caring responses.

If you have a fussy or unpredictable baby, you may begin to worry about bonding and attachment. How can you have a close, secure attachment when you don't feel confident in your ability to calm and soothe your baby? Those early moments of joy and connection may feel like a distant memory, especially if you spend most of your waking hours caring for a crying baby. Your idea of a good day may entail one in which you are actually able to get dressed and brush your teeth! When you don't have time for a break and self-care feels like a luxury you cannot afford, it can be easy to lose perspective. You may be putting in hard work but lacking those rewarding moments of interaction with your baby. If the stress takes an even greater toll, you may begin to lose hope and to feel like you are failing as a new parent.

Fortunately, we are learning a great deal more about the attachment process and how parent-baby attachment evolves and is protected. The most reassuring fact is that babies are tougher than we might realize, and they have the ability to recover from difficult experiences. This is a quality called *resilience*. It means that your baby can tolerate both bad and good experiences, and she is able to attach to more than 1 person. If you have a spouse or partner, grandparents, and/or nannies and other caregivers, there will be more sources of support to shape your baby's emotional development. No parent should worry that he or she is on his or her own with such a heavy responsibility.

Attachment: Why Is It Important?

Attachment refers to a relationship that emerges over time and is based on a deep emotional connection between baby and caregiver(s). As you care for and interact with your baby during the first year, she will respond and organize her behavior around you and around other consistent caregivers.

Did You Know?

The term *attachment* emerged from extensive research and studies that took place in the 1960s and 1970s, mostly conducted by 2 researchers, John Bowlby and Mary Ainsworth. From their extensive study of parent-baby interactions, they developed and refined a definition for attachment.

All newborns have instinctual attachment behaviors that trigger in response to different needs and emotional states. These include vocalizing or crying, grasping, moving, and sucking. When and how you respond to these behaviors affects how your baby develops. Over time, the process of attachment depends on interactions where you and your baby learn to relate to each other in predictable patterns. You both play an important role in building patterns of interactions, and these patterns become strengthened with repetition and consistency. If your baby shows fewer predictable behaviors, you may find it challenging to know how to respond, and you might also start to doubt your skills. Similarly, if you are not able to consistently respond to specific cues, your baby may stop exhibiting them. Consider the following scenarios and how you might respond:

Scenario #1: A baby wakes up after a 2-hour nap and begins to cry and fuss. Dad picks her up, soothes her, and then changes her diaper. She calms briefly but then begins to cry again. Dad prepares a bottle and feeds her. The baby accepts the bottle and remains quiet but awake upon finishing it.

Scenario #2: A baby who has been awake begins to cry. Mom begins breastfeeding. The baby latches briefly but then pulls off. He continues to cry while mom attempts to hold and rock him. As he becomes more upset, mom again tries to feed him without success. She finally lays him down in his crib. He calms briefly but quickly starts crying again. Mom checks his diaper and sees that he is wet. After a change, he remains calm for a brief period but then fusses again. This time, he breastfeeds and falls asleep while feeding.

Scenario #3: New parents bring their baby to a family party. The baby is very fussy, and so they try to feed her. She isn't able to feed for more than a brief period, and her eyes dart around the room. After a while, she pushes the bottle away and cries. Her parents are sure she is hungry, so they continue to offer the bottle. Numerous other family members offer to hold and feed her, but this only makes her more upset. When it becomes clear she is not going to settle, her parents leave the party, and she falls asleep on the ride home.

All these scenarios include possible "miscommunications" between baby and caregiver, but they turn out differently. Before placing blame on yourself or any caregiver(s) for these types of occurrences, keep in mind the challenges that different babies might present. As you learned in Chapter 4, babies differ in their ability to give clear and predictable signals to their caregivers. Additionally, a new or different environment can affect how your baby's signals are expressed and how you are able to make sense of them. Even if your baby is predictable, you should feel reassured to know that trial and error is a normal process, and it won't last forever. Remember to keep perspective, even in the toughest moments. Who doesn't recall a family party that ended in disaster? Or a road trip that seemed like it would never end? As devoted parents, you try to respond to your baby's stress as best you can. If you learn from these experiences, they can add immense value to your bag of tricks, and your confidence will begin to emerge. Perhaps you learned that movement from the car helped your baby to fall asleep easily. Or you gained insight about the importance of finding a quiet room when it is time to nurse. Thus, these dreaded miscommunications can become learning moments between parents and babies. Even if you've had the worst possible experience and can't think of 1 new skill you learned, know that it's OK! With more time and experience, you and your baby will learn to adapt, and your attachment relationship will be preserved.

Let's talk in more detail about attachment and why it is so important. When your baby has a secure attachment to you, she begins to experience trust. Other benefits of attachment include

- Trust becomes the expectation for her future relationships, allowing for other meaningful relationships to be formed.
- The effect of stressful experiences is reduced.
- Your baby feels secure to actively explore her environment, leading her to develop intellectually and socially and become more independent as she moves and plays.
- Emotional development is supported as your baby learns to manage her emotions and behavior.
- A sense of identify begins to form.

Attachment Development

Attachment behaviors can be observed by the time your baby is 6 to 8 weeks of age when she begins to show slight preferences for specific caregivers. For instance, she may prefer being held by her dad because he is with her for more hours of the day and his touch feels more familiar. Or she may fuss when her grandmother comes to see her and takes her from her mother's familiar arms. If your baby nurses, she is likely to prefer her mother because she is able to sense both the comfort and nourishment that she has come to trust. These preferences will begin to emerge during this developmental period. However, the most important task for your very young baby is learning how to give signals (eg, crying, fussing) that will attract any caregiver to respond (eg, mother, father, grandparent, babysitter).

Between 2 and 6 months of age, your baby will continue to develop more ways to communicate wants and needs, and she will also get better at recognizing familiar and unfamiliar adults and caregivers. At this stage, your baby may begin to show more significant preferences. This might include preferring you over your partner or preferring either of you over a less familiar or new caregiver. If your baby is fussy, she may show these preferences more strongly, especially if you are better able than your partner to read her cues and provide the soothing responses that she needs. Perhaps the reverse is true, and you are noticing that your baby consistently seems to prefer your partner. While this can feel disheartening, you should know that you are not alone! While this might feel like a rejection, these early months with your baby are only the start of the attachment relationship. With patience and persistence, you can develop new skills along with your baby. Your partner or spouse can also be a source of support by sharing the strategies that he or she has mastered in interactions with your baby. It's so important to stay involved and to trust that your efforts will be rewarded!

Around 7 to 8 months of age, the attachment relationship between you and your baby becomes even stronger. By this age, your baby will exhibit a strong preference for you and your partner. Now that she recognizes other familiar caregivers such as extended family or babysitters, she may develop preferences among this group of people. Your baby is also making great strides in her cognitive skills, and this allows her to begin to process new information. For instance, she will soon grasp the idea of *object permanence*. Object permanence refers to babies' ability to learn that when they cannot see or hear something, it does not mean that the object or person has disappeared. In simpler terms, babies are aware that you exist, even when you are not present! It makes sense that this would be the age when separation anxiety develops. Now that your baby has a strong attachment and can remember you when you are absent, she will become more upset about being separated. She may also become cautious of new or unfamiliar people. This is commonly known as *stranger anxiety*.

Between 9 and 12 months of age, your baby has strong emotional bonds to a second parent and to other familiar individuals such as grandparents and siblings. While multiple attachments are forming, it's still typical for your baby to exhibit preferences and to be inconsistent in her reactions. For instance, a breastfed baby will naturally seek her mother when she is hungry but may prefer to play with her father or older sister. She may sometimes cry when her dad leaves the house but not react in other instances. Similarly, someone new coming into the home may cause a baby to immediately seek her mother, but she may be less bothered by a room full of strangers when she goes into a new and interesting environment. Your baby's reactions can be influenced by many other things, such as feeling hungry or tired, and she may also respond differently if she is distracted or overwhelmed.

Separation Anxiety

Your baby may show different degrees of separation anxiety and cautiousness with new people well into her second year. You should not feel alarmed if your baby seems anxious when separating from you. This is a typical response. Learning to cope with separation is an important part of the attachment process for both you and your baby. As your baby gets more practice separating from you and then being reunited, she will develop an important new sense of trust and confidence in her attachment relationship. She also will have the opportunity to accept caregiving and direction from other adults, which has many benefits. For instance, exposure to new caregivers and environments may help your baby to develop more flexibility in how she copes with stress. She may also have new learning experiences as she explores a novel environment. Your baby will also expand her social skills by learning to engage and relate to new caregivers and peers.

While it may be stressful to watch your baby go through difficult separation experiences, keep in mind that avoiding separation is not the answer! This can often lead to more challenges as your baby continues to grow and develop. If your baby does not separate frequently from you, she may not develop important skills for building relationships with others and coping with stress. She may not feel secure enough to explore the world around her and to engage with other adults and children. This can slow progress with other skills such as movement, play, and cognitive skill development. It can also lead to persistent feelings of anxiety and insecurity when faced with any type of new challenge.

Understanding the importance of your baby learning to cope with separations may help you feel less anxious about these experiences. If you are working on separation, it's important to pay attention to how you are feeling. If you are struggling during this time but your baby is responding well, this is good news! It means that your baby has formed a healthy attachment relationship with you. Of course, it's natural for you to feel conflicted about leaving your baby. While these feelings can be upsetting, they will improve with more time and practice. What's most important is trying to manage your emotional responses as best you can. Babies are very perceptive. If you feel nervous or hesitant about leaving your baby with another caregiver, your baby may begin to notice your feelings and may display more emotional responses. By contrast, if you can show a calm and positive demeanor, your baby will respond better to separations, eventually showing less distress and more curiosity about new people and environments. Remember that separation is a skill for both of you, and it can be developed with practice.

For parents who have concern for separation anxiety, there are many enjoyable games and activities that can improve both you and your baby's comfort level with separation. For the young baby, this can begin with the familiar and fun activity known as peek-a-boo. Your baby will start to trust that you are still behind the blanket or towel. As your baby becomes mobile, this can be expanded into games like hide-and-seek. Have your baby try to "find" you in different rooms of the house. You can also hide toys and other fun objects and then help your baby to locate them. Keep it fun but also safe by never leaving your baby unsupervised. For the older baby, you can "practice" separation by leaving her frequently with another caregiver but for very short periods of time (approximately 2–5 minutes). You can gradually increase the duration of these separations as your baby becomes more comfortable with your absence. Make your departure quick but positive by always saying good-bye (avoid advice from friends that it is best to "sneak out," as this can cause your baby to feel more distrustful). If your baby is distressed, don't linger and make the parting even more emotional. This will likely increase stress for both of you! Remember, the more opportunities your baby has to practice separation, the more likely she is to feel confident knowing that you will return. Don't wait until the day before returning to work to address concerns with separation!

Types of Attachment

A secure attachment affords babies many positive benefits as they grow and develop. But what happens when attachments are not secure? In trying to answer this question, it's important to understand the different types of attachment relationships and how they might be influenced. Research on attachment styles examined interactions between parents and babies 12 to 18 months of age. Babies were observed playing alone with a parent, then observed after their parent briefly left the room, and then again after the parent returned. Results from these studies revealed 3 primary attachment styles, as well as a fourth style that was identified later in studies of young children exposed to abuse and/or trauma. Following are brief descriptions of the 3 primary styles observed in 12- to 18-month-olds:

Secure

This attachment style is the most common (and best!). These babies are able to move away from their parent and actively explore, but they periodically approach or look to their parent for reassurance. While they show immediate distress when their parent leaves the room, they seek their parent for comfort when he or she returns, and they are easily soothed. Babies with secure attachment are able to quickly recover and begin to play again.

Insecure-Avoidant

Babies with this attachment style may also separate easily to explore their environment, but they do not necessarily seek out their parent while playing. When the parent leaves the room, these babies may not have any emotional reaction, and they may also not react when a parent returns to the room. If they become distressed, they may not approach their parent for reassurance.

Insecure-Ambivalent/Resistant

These babies have difficulty moving away from their parent to explore and play. They may cling to their mother or father, showing distress in a new environment. These babies become quite distressed when the parent leaves the room. However, when the parent returns, they are often not easily soothed by efforts made by the parent. Thus, they show an ambivalent behavioral style by resisting separation, yet later rejecting their parent when they try to reconnect and offer comfort and interaction.

A fourth attachment style was added many years after the original research that identified these 3 primary styles. The fourth style, called *disorganized,* was identified to describe attachment behaviors in infants who have likely been exposed to neglect, abuse, and/or trauma. In these cases, the parent's behavior might be unpredictable. As a result, no organized strategy for attachment works consistently for the baby, and so the baby's responses do not follow any type of consistent pattern. The baby may respond with fear toward a parent in one instance and then seek the parent and cling to him or her in another situation. Because this attachment style is less understood and believed to occur primarily in infants exposed to extreme circumstances, it requires attention from skilled professionals to understand fearful and conflicted responses. (If you suspect your baby has experienced abuse, neglect, or trauma, you should immediately bring this concern to your pediatrician, who can assist with referrals for appropriate follow-up.)

Babies with a secure attachment style can use their parent as a "home base" from which to move and explore. They have great trust in the caregiving relationship because most of their early experiences have been positive; their needs have been understood and met. For babies with insecure attachments, this sense of trust will not be as strong. As a result, separations might be more stressful for the baby, and they may not easily respond to efforts made by the parent to offer comfort. It's important to understand why insecure attachments might form and what you can do if you are worried about an insecure attachment with your baby.

Attachment Concerns

Most babies naturally form secure attachments to 1 or more caregivers during their first year. However, about 30% of babies show features of an anxious or insecure attachment between 1 and 2 years of age. *Anxious* or *insecure attachment* refers to avoidant or ambivalent patterns of relating to their parent/caregiver shown by some babies. Although this percentage might seem alarmingly high, especially if you are experiencing challenges with a fussy baby, there is important information you should understand.

- Insecure attachment is associated with many different risk factors, and most are unrelated to fussiness.
- Insecure attachment is not the same as an *attachment disorder,* which is characterized by a disorganized attachment style. Attachment disorders are rare, and they develop in children who have experienced extremely poor care such as ongoing neglect, being deprived of basic needs related to comfort and stimulation, and not having any consistent caregiver during the first years. In most cases, these are children who have been reared in institutions or under other extremely adverse circumstances.
- Insecure attachment does not necessarily result in future adjustment problems. In fact, most babies with attachment concerns do not grow up to have significant behavioral or emotional problems, especially if they do not have other risk factors such as the ones described in the following sections.

Consider the following additional information, which describes other situations and risk factors that may contribute to attachment concerns in young babies. Some of these concerns relate to you as a parent, some to the environment, and some to your baby.

Parent/Environment

Difficulties in the environment can affect attachment. Living in poverty, being homeless or having an unstable or unsafe home environment, exposure to abuse and/or neglect, and conflict between parents are associated with higher levels of insecure attachment relationships. Another important risk factor is when 1 or both parents experiences personal problems or mental illness, especially if it is not being treated appropriately. *Mental illness* commonly refers to anxiety or mood disorders, but it also includes substance misuse, addictions, post-traumatic stress disorder, and a host of other concerns. While some individuals cope successfully with mental illness and simultaneously care for a baby, many others experience significant challenges that affect every part of their life, including daily routines, employment, and maintaining relationships with family and friends.

In many cases, risk factors coincide. For example, a parent who is living in poverty may also experience a mental illness such as depression and find it challenging to obtain employment. When there are many challenges, attachment development is affected in different ways. In some instances, parents have less time to spend with their baby because of their need to work. This results in fewer opportunities for parent and baby to interact and gain familiarity with each other. Even when parents are physically present, if they feel overwhelmed or significantly distracted, they might be unable to respond in the predictable patterns that support healthy attachment. While family support can buffer the effect of these situations, it may not be available for all new parents. Fortunately, there are resources available in many communities intended to support young families, especially those that might be at higher risk for different adjustment problems.

The Infant Personality

A successful relationship between you and your baby not only depends on your background and issues but also on the personality of your baby. A baby's personality, or temperament, which emerges at birth, contributes greatly to parent-baby attachment. Babies who exhibit an *easy* temperament are more likely to develop secure attachments. These babies respond positively to new experiences, are easily soothed, and readily establish predictable patterns with regard to eating and sleeping. Babies who are *slow to warm up* exhibit anxious responses, take longer to establish regular sleep and feeding patterns, and require more parental support to adapt to new things. Babies with *difficult* temperament are the most challenging to a parent. These babies do not establish regular sleep or feeding patterns, often react negatively to new people and experiences, and have difficulty soothing and adapting to their environments. Babies in the latter 2 categories may be at higher risk for anxious attachment, but this is only 1 piece of the puzzle. Most experts agree that it is a combination of factors that shapes development of the attachment relationship; babies present with certain personality traits, and parent(s) must learn respond to them. If you are worried that your baby has a difficult temperament, you should know that this does not mean your attachment will be insecure. With extra patience and persistence, it is very possible to develop a secure attachment.

Recovering From Stress

A parent's ability to recover from negative experiences, a process known as *resilience,* is just as important. Pay attention to your feelings and personal challenges. If you recognize that you have extra stress in your life that affects your ability to provide consistent and loving care for your baby, it's crucial that you seek appropriate help. This is *not* an admission of failure. Quite the opposite—it's the first courageous step toward protecting your relationship with your baby. New parents should expect that they will have successes and make mistakes as they learn to care for their baby. Parents must also develop resilience skills by recognizing their needs and seeking the right support.

Even without significant sources of extra stress, it's still quite normal to feel exhausted, overwhelmed, and depleted as a new parent. A short break can offer much-needed time to recharge, even if this means only a handful of deep breaths between efforts to calm and soothe a fussy baby. In a 2-parent household, sharing the caregiving duties can allow for both parents to have support, breaks, and shared opportunities for bonding. While not every baby has 2 available parents/caregivers, remember that babies can attach to more than 1 person. Allowing your baby to spend regular time with other caregivers is a wonderful way to extend their social and emotional experiences while allowing you some time to take care of yourself.

Most importantly, look for moments between naps and feedings when your baby is calm and alert and so are you. It might be tempting to grab this downtime to complete other chores. While these moments might be fleeting and short-lived (especially with a fussy baby), they can also be the most rewarding opportunities of the day, to simply watch, be with, and enjoy your baby! Allowing special time for bonding, when you have no other demands, can help you reconnect with the joy of being a parent and strengthen the unique emotional connection you share with your baby.

Seeking Help

If reading this information causes you to recognize possible signs of an insecure attachment with your baby, or if you have concerns that you or your partner may need additional support or mental health treatment, consider seeking guidance and input from a qualified health care professional. Talking with your pediatrician can be the best place to start. Your doctor can listen to your concerns and determine what type of professional is best to consult. This may include a psychologist with expertise in infant development and mental health, a counselor or therapist who understands adult mental health or adjustment issues, or a combination of providers who can evaluate both you and your baby. In many cases, this includes additional education, counseling, evaluation of your baby's development, and identification of appropriate resources. Even if no concerns are identified, you may feel empowered with additional support and insights and also reassured that you've taken the right steps for both you and your baby!

A Strong, Trusting Relationship

Babies naturally form attachments to their parents and close caregivers. The process is ongoing, and dynamic; you and your baby both engage and respond to each other. Most babies form secure attachments based on positive caregiving experiences, and this leads to a strong, trusting relationship. While it's normal to worry about attachment when you have a fussy baby, keep in mind that the attachment process is based on many months and literally thousands of interactions between you and your baby. No parent gets it right responding to a baby's needs every single time! Working through and resolving these "misunderstandings" are a natural part of the attachment process. Each time, you build new skills, confidence, and trust, while strengthening your attachment bond. Babies also learn from these experiences; they adjust their attachment-seeking behaviors and develop new skills for adapting to stress. This process of resilience supports attachment, allowing a baby to tolerate and recover from stressful experiences and, eventually, to separate and practice independence skills. While it's true that "easy" babies recover more quickly and develop skills more readily than others, it's the underlying emotional connection and persistence that keeps the attachment relationship warm and thriving.

Chapter 8

A Calming Touch: Baby Massage

Touch is critical to creating attachment between parents and their baby and is an important sensation throughout life. Research has shown that a baby feels touch at different stages of development while in utero. Skin-to-skin touch is very important; right after delivery, the doctor will place the baby on the mother's body, providing immediate skin-to-skin sensory input. The baby may start to "crawl" to the breast and root to the breast in direct response to the touch (or *tactile*) sensory system.

Communicating Love

Touch communicates love. It sends wordless messages of sympathy and security—with your baby, with your significant other, and with friends and family. You hug someone after an absence; you pat their back or give a high five for a job well done. You hold a friend's hand for support, give a backrub to a significant other to soothe stress, or gently stroke your partner's hair back when he or she is crying.

Touch with babies can include many things, such as holding, stroking, cuddling, patting, kissing, caressing, breastfeeding, skin-to-skin contact, and baby massage. These comforting touches have an extremely positive effect on the physical and emotional development of your baby, and you can provide all of them repeatedly throughout the day. (Remember, dads or partners can provide these touch experiences as well as mothers!) Some therapists call this deep touch pressure, and research shows that deep touch pressure has a calming and organizing effect on the nervous system. Deep touch pressure is considered firm, gentle, consistent pressure on the body. It positively affects the autonomic nervous system, which regulates breathing and heart rate. Deep touch pressure taps into our touch system but also the proprioceptive system. (See Chapter 5.) Babies respond differently to deep touch pressure, so make sure to read your baby's cues to see if he likes it or not. If he does not like the touch, hold the body part firmly without moving your hands. Then, as tolerated, you can slowly move your hands while maintaining the firm pressure.

Did You Know?

In the neonatal intensive care unit, babies are given skin-to-skin contact with their parents/caregivers if they are medically stable. This is called *kangaroo care*, and it involves placing the baby on a parent's chest and wrapping a blanket around both, mirroring a mother kangaroo holding a baby kangaroo in her pouch. The benefits of kangaroo care are numerous for both baby (for physiological stability) and parent (for bonding and confidence).

Using deep touch pressure helps to calm and organize your baby, which helps to create positive touch experiences. The following CALM touch strategies do not have to be done all at once; nor do they have to be in a certain order. Simply use these strategies throughout the day. Both mom and dad can provide this input. Some specific CALM touch strategies you can try with your baby include

Back: Use deep touch pressure down the back. Use firm pressure and move from your baby's shoulders down to his lower back. You can do this to help increase his tolerance of tummy time. You can also just put your hand firmly on your baby's bottom while he is on his tummy to help support him in this position (see Chapter 12 for more information on this and different holds and carries that involve deep touch pressure). You can also do this firm pressure down your baby's back while you are holding him in different positions on your lap, while he is sitting independently, or when he is being cradled in your arms.

Hands: Touch and firmly hold your baby's hands. Put your thumb in her palm and hold your fingers down on the top of her hand. You can bring her hands together or do 1 hand at a time. You can also massage the palm of her hand in a circular motion. This really helps if your baby tends to keep her hands fisted.

Feet: Touch and firmly hold your baby's feet, one in each hand. Gently clap his feet together to provide more input. For a foot massage, hold the ankle in 1 hand and use your free hand to hold the foot with your fingers on top and thumb underneath. Stroke firmly along the foot and gently tug on the toes. Make sure to use deep touch pressure; if you stroke too lightly, it will tickle him.

Shoulders: Rub her shoulders while she sits supported on your lap and firmly move your hands down her arms. Who does not like a little shoulder rub at times?

Body: When she is on her back, firmly touch down her body. Start at the head and move along the outside of her body all the way down to her feet. You can also move your hands down the center of her body; start at the chest and move toward the belly, and down the front of her legs.

Head: Some babies love having their head stroked, and some babies don't, so watch your baby's reaction! Cup your hands around your baby's head and stroke him simultaneously backwards over the crown of his head. Stroke along the jawline and bring your hands toward the chin. Stroke across the forehead and across the eyebrows. You can also do small circles on his cheeks and squeeze the chin. Figure out what touch your baby likes on his face and do any or all of these.

You can incorporate massage and deep touch pressure with your baby into everyday care, such as baths or diaper changes, soothing your baby to sleep, calming and readying your baby for a feeding, or during playtime—almost any time! Here are some key points.

- After a bath, wrap your baby in a towel and run some long, firm strokes down her arms, legs, and back.
- During diaper changes provide a little tummy massage. (See The Colic Relief Routine section later in this chapter.)
- Touch and hold a baby's foot during a fussy time or during a feeding—just make sure your baby tolerates it well and that it helps soothe her!

The benefits of massage have been known for a long time with adults and have been studied more recently with preterm, fussy, and typically developing babies. Research with preterm babies shows positive effects of massage in the neonatal intensive care unit, including better digestion and weight gain. Asian, African, and Indian cultures have used massage in their care of babies for centuries and understand the benefits of touch.

"

"Learning to massage my baby has really helped me be more comfortable with handling her. I felt awkward before because I had not held many babies prior to having my own. Now I understand her body more so we both feel more at ease when I am holding her."

Father of an 8-week-old fussy baby

"

Benefits of Touch Pressure and Massage

Deep touch pressure and massage are now more important than ever. Parents today use more baby-holding equipment than in the past, such as bouncy seats, swings, walkers, and jumpers. As more and more pieces of equipment are available on the market today, parents buy them thinking they must need them. Pediatric physical therapists have labeled this generation "container babies" or "bucket babies" because they may be in containers more than in someone's arms or on the floor to play. Babies are often in these pieces of equipment too long throughout the day. Therapists also talk about the "container shuffle," which is when parents move their babies from container to container—the swing, the bouncy chair, the car seat—throughout the day. (See Chapter 12 on postural control and the disadvantages of using this equipment.) The benefits of holding, carrying, wearing, and handling your baby supersede the benefits of these pieces of equipment and cannot be overstated. Some people describe this generation as a "high tech and low touch" world. Make sure positive touch experiences are a part of your baby's world.

One of the first things we teach parents of fussy babies is the calming power of touch. We start with gentle stroking and deep touch pressure and move toward baby massage as babies tolerate touch. Massage strokes are simple but so powerful in what they do for your baby.

Emotional and Psychological Benefits

Baby massage has emotional and psychological benefits, such as

- Gaining confidence in handling your baby
- Learning to read your baby's cues—what he likes and doesn't like— through nonverbal communication

- Promoting engagement and intimacy with your baby
- Creating a positive interaction between you and your baby, leading to bonding and attachment
- Calming and relaxing both you and your baby through 1-on-1 quality time with your little one
- Building trust between you and your baby (He will learn to feel secure.)
- Promoting a connection between your baby's mind and body
- Communicating a message of love (It helps you and your baby fall in love!)

Physical and Physiological Benefits

Baby massage also has physical and physiological benefits, such as

- Increases newborn sleep organization
- Helps your baby calm down and lowers the level of cortisol (the stress hormone)
- Helps your baby relax and get ready for sleep
- Leads to flexibility of the arms and legs as it relaxes the muscles
- Helps with digestion
- Helps with constipation
- Reduces colic symptoms of irritability, especially when you do the Colic Relief Routine (See later in this chapter.)
- Helps with circulation
- Boosts your baby's immune system
- With oil, helps with dry skin
- Decreases your baby's skin sensitivity
- Raises a baby's stimulation threshold
- Aids in respiration
- Promotes good body awareness for your baby

A Positive Touch Experience

During a massage, learn to interpret your baby's reaction to touch by watching his body language. This helps you learn how to read his cues (see Chapter 4). While mothers experience intimate physical contact when breastfeeding, fathers and partners can use massage for that important skin-to-skin contact. There is no right or wrong way to massage your baby; it is just a positive touch experience. It is also a wonderful way for dads to make a connection with their babies. Research has shown that dads who massage their babies are more involved in their day-to-day care. Massaging colicky or fussy babies is a wonderful experience, and parents often report that it helps them feel like they are doing something positive with and for their babies.

Baby Massage Resources

For a great resource to learn massage, go to www.infantmassageusa.org, find a Certified Educator of Infant Massage near you, and sign up for the 4- to 6-week session class. In these classes, you will learn the benefits of massage, what oils to use, the best position for you to massage your baby, how to ask for permission to do massage, what type of pressure you use for the strokes, when and where you should massage, and the entire baby massage protocol. You can also find various online videos that teach massage, but before watching any, ensure that it is led by a person certified to teach massage to parents.

At the beginning, some babies take a little longer to get used to the massage, especially sensitive babies. Don't give up! Try to do the massage for several days in a row. You may not get through the entire baby massage protocol, but at least do parts of it. The entire protocol includes massage strokes for the legs, tummy, chest, arms, back, and face. The best time to massage your baby is when he is in the quiet alert state. Read his cues; your baby will let you know when the best time is to do his massage. You can also try doing the massage when your baby is in the active alert or fussy state, as this may help move him to the quiet alert state. However, if he seems overstimulated or uncomfortable and starts to cry, stop and try again at another time. Some parents love to include massage as a part of their nighttime routine; however, with some babies it is too alerting right before bed, so, again, watch your baby's cues. If your baby doesn't like a certain stroke, you can use a technique called *touch and hold*. This is when you touch and hold a body part firmly, so your baby gets used to you touching that body part. You may get to a certain point in the massage and he starts fussing; it may just be that at that certain point, he's had enough and met his sensory threshold! This does not necessarily mean that he doesn't like that certain body part massaged. If he does fuss at a certain point just try starting at a different body part for the next massage. Watch your baby's cues and let him tell you what he likes best.

Once you learn the entire massage protocol, try to massage your baby once a day. But don't feel guilty if you can't get it done every day; it is still beneficial even a couple times a week. It is wonderful for both mom and dad to learn the massage, as their touch is different, and you can take turns providing this lovely experience. Grandparents love to massage their grandbabies, so teach them as well. Teaching massage to your child care provider is not recommended; this is an intimate touch experience that is best provided by parents or other trusted caregivers.

Many parents have positive comments on the benefits of the massage for mom, dad, and baby.

> "My day is so busy that taking time to massage my baby makes me feel like I am doing something that my baby really enjoys, and I love it too!"
>
> Parent of a 4-week-old baby

The Colic Relief Routine

The Colic Relief Routine is something I (Patti) recommend to all parents of fussy or colicky babies. Derived from Vimala McClure, founder of the International Association of Infant Massage and author of *Infant Massage: A Handbook for Loving Parents*, McClure found the great benefit massage has for fussy babies. Parents report that this routine does bring relief to their fussy baby. There are 7 parts to the Colic Relief Routine. If your baby does not tolerate this massage, use touch relaxation (page 82) while he gets used to you touching his tummy. It is ideal to do this while he is in the quiet alert state and wait for at least 30 minutes after eating before trying. It can also help to release gas, so try it when he is a little fussy—but if he gets fussier, stop! Don't do this routine or any massage while your baby is asleep.

You can do the Colic Relief Routine with the baby's clothes on or off with some oil. Oil helps your hands move smoothly over your baby's stomach. Use a natural oil like grape-seed, sunflower, or olive. It is not recommended to use adult massage oils, hand lotion, or nut-based oils due to possible allergies. Do these 7 steps 3 times through at least 2 times a day.

1. **Resting hands.** Resting hands (Figure 8.1) communicates to your baby that you are ready to start a tummy massage; he will learn to relax. Rest your hands on your baby's tummy, relaxing yourself completely even if your baby is fussing and crying. You can verbally "ask him for permission" to do the massage, which is *your* cue to him about what is coming!

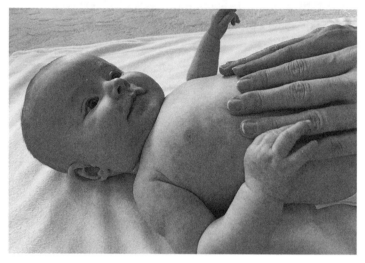

Figure 8.1. Resting hands.

2. **Water wheel.** Make paddling strokes on your baby's tummy, one hand following the other, as if you were scooping a depression into sand (Figure 8.2). Keep your hands molded to your baby's tummy. Do not use the edge of your hand. Make sure you stay below the rib cage. Repeat 6 times.

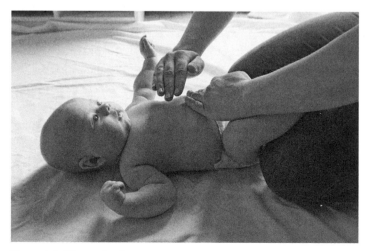

Figure 8.2. Water wheel.

3. **Up down.** Push your baby's knees together up into the tummy and
   gently push into his tummy (Figure 8.3), and then stretch your baby's
   knees out straight. Make sure the knees are together, so the top of the
   legs touches his tummy. Don't have them out to the side of his body, as
   you won't get any pressure on the stomach. Hold for about 6 seconds.
   If the baby resists by straightening his legs, bounce his legs gently and
   encourage him to relax.

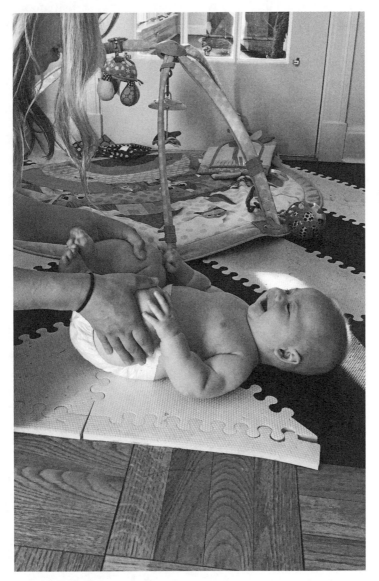

Figure 8.3. Up down.

4. **Touch relaxation.** This is a conditioned response that helps your baby relax; you can use this at other times during the day. Gently release the pressure from the previous stroke, then stroke his legs downward to coax him to release tension and relax.

5. **Sun moon.** This is the trickiest stroke to learn, but you'll get the hang of it. Start on the baby's right side under his rib cage. Begin with your left hand and stroke in a full circle, moving clockwise (Figure 8.4). As your left hand is making the lower part of the circle, make a half moon with your right hand (Figure 8.5), just below the rib cage, stroking in the same direction. It is important to remember that both hands move in the same clockwise direction continuously as you move along the colon.

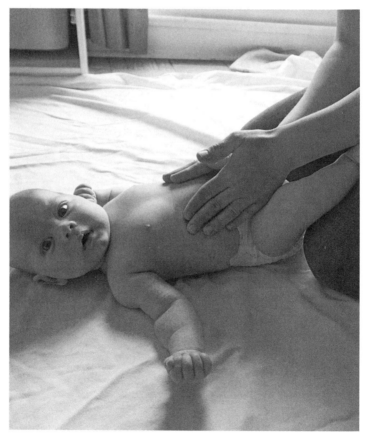

Figure 8.4. Sun moon. (This is the beginning of the sun moon stroke when the left hand circles around the stomach.)

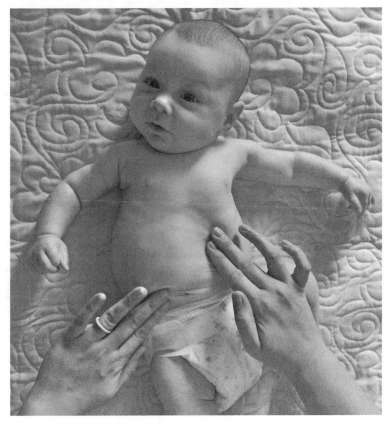

Figure 8.5. Sun moon. (This is the end of the sun moon stroke when the right hand moves across the top of the stomach under the rib cage in a half-moon stroke.)

6. **Up down.** This is the same as stroke 3—second time around.
7. **Touch relaxation.** This is the same as stroke 4—second time around.

It may take several days for your baby to tolerate this sequence and to show the benefits, such as expelling gas or moving the bowels. During the routine, remember to count the strokes and hold your baby's knees up to a count of 6. Hearing your voice and feeling the touch of your hands may help your baby relax. Some parents see immediate results with gas relief; other parents feel it helps a little. Try it twice a day for at least 2 weeks. During this time, don't worry about doing the entire baby massage protocol; that may take too much time. If you don't see a change, your baby may not be that gassy, but it is definitely worth a try.

Massage: A Positive Effect

Massaging your baby expresses your love to him and helps you build a warm and wonderful relationship. Baby massage is about being together physically and emotionally with moms and dads. There is a short window of time that you can massage your baby; once he starts crawling, he will be on the go, and it's harder to do the entire massage. But if you start the massage soon after birth, he will have learned the calming power of touch.

> "*Doing the Colic Relief Routine made such a difference with my baby's fussiness. I felt like it really relieved his gas pain. He was happier every time I did it!*"
>
> Mother of an 8-week-old baby

Chapter 9

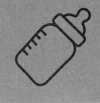

The Secret of Sleep

Whoever said, "I slept like a baby," did not have a fussy baby who didn't sleep well! Sleep is a precious commodity, and lack of sleep is detrimental in many ways for both parent and baby. A big concern we hear from parents of fussy babies is that their baby's sleep is "horrible." They may get all sorts of advice from families and friends about what to do. There are also hundreds of resources, social media posts, blogs, and books about baby sleep, all with varied theories that may be at polar opposites. It may feel almost impossible to figure out what will work for you and your baby!

This chapter offers an overview of baby sleep focusing on birth to 6 months of age and covers topics such as

- Normal sleep
- The importance of sleep
- Safe sleep practices
- Typical sleep issues with fussy babies
- Setting the stage for good sleep throughout your baby's lifetime
- How and why to sleep train

This chapter cannot be as comprehensive as some of the books dedicated solely to sleep. There are numerous well-written books on sleep that are extremely thorough and are great references on pediatric sleep in general (see Resources).

A Baby's Normal Sleep Patterns

To understand poor sleep, let's first take a look at what normal sleep is. As we learned in Chapter 6, there are 2 sleep states, quiet or deep sleep and active or light sleep. Drowsiness is another state of arousal, which is a transitional state from awake to sleeping or sleeping to awake. In normal sleep, adults and babies move through sleep cycles—different levels or states of sleep—throughout the night and during some naps. A normal sleep cycle transitions from drowsiness to active sleep, into quiet sleep, and then back into active sleep again. An adult's sleep cycle lasts about 90 minutes, while a baby's cycle is about 45 to 50 minutes. Babies usually spend 10 to 15 minutes in active sleep, then are in quiet sleep for the next 20 to 25 minutes, and then are back to active sleep for another 10 to 15 minutes. This means more than half of their sleep time is in active sleep! Deep sleep is critical for everyone but especially fussy babies because often they don't get to a nice deep sleep. Deep sleep is very important to "recharge" your baby's brain, which allows more learning to happen in the awake time. Sleep-wake cycles are strongly affected by hunger and feeding during the first 2 months of age as babies get hungry, eat, and fall asleep several times throughout the day.

Typical Sleep in Babies

Table 9.1 summarizes some general information about sleep. The point of this chart is for you to get an idea of how much sleep is really needed at different ages. Despite these being guidelines, this chart provides insight into what is typical and what to strive for.

As previously mentioned, Table 9.1 is only a guideline. There is a lot of variability from baby to baby, so don't worry if your baby is not getting the exact number of hours listed in the chart. Sleep duration also varies day to day with babies and what occurs in their environment. Parents hear of all the long-term effects of sleep deprivation in adults and often worry about sleep deprivation in babies, but it doesn't pertain to young babies. If you are concerned about how little sleep your baby receives (or if you think he sleeps too much), keep track for a couple days and share the information with your pediatrician. You can use the Behavior Diary in Resources to keep track. (See "Sleep Challenges for Fussy Babies" box later in this chapter.)

At 0 to 2 weeks of age, there isn't much difference between daytime and nighttime sleep, as newborns sleep most of the 24 hours in a day. But by 5 to 6 weeks of age, babies begin to show a day-night sleep cycle, which

Table 9.1. Average Hours of Sleep for Babies

Age	Naps	Total Nap Hours	Stretches of Sleep	Total Night Sleep Hours[a]	Average Total for 24 h
0–4 wk	Variable and many	7–9 h	Variable One 4- to 5-h stretch at night Multiple 2- to 4-h stretches of daytime sleep	7–9 h	18–20 h
1–2 mo	3–5	5–7 h	One 6- to 7-h stretch at night 2- to 4-h naps	8–10 h	16–18 h
3–5 mo	3–4	3–5 h	One 8- to 10-h stretch at night 3- to 4-h naps	9.5–12 h	14–18 h
6–8 mo	3	3–4 h	One 8- to 10-h stretch at night 3- to 4-h naps	10–12 h	14–15 h

[a] This can be 2 stretches of sleep, 1 long stretch and 1 shorter stretch of sleep.

has longer stretches of sleep at night and more wakefulness during the day. Remember that when we talk about stretches of sleep, babies are cycling through active and quiet sleep. They are not in one sleep state for very long. This means the 6-hour stretch is not just quiet sleep but a combination of quiet and active sleep. At 6 to 12 weeks of age, babies may have one 6- to 7-hour stretch of sleep at night, which may delay that first night feeding—so you get a little more sleep! These longer stretches of sleep may kick in at different times; some babies fall asleep at 10:00 pm, while some night owls stay up until 1:00 or 2:00 am. Remember, all babies are different! Focus on picking up your baby's pattern, and you'll learn what to expect. The more regular rhythms of sleepiness and alertness generally develop between 2 and 4 months, but each baby will develop at her own pace.

In the sleep study world, people often say, "Sleep begets sleep." What does that mean? It means the more a baby sleeps, the more a baby will sleep. Research shows that the better a baby naps during the day, the better she sleeps at night. Parents often try to keep their baby up during the day, thinking this will help with nighttime sleep, but it doesn't work that way. Nighttime sleep is usually worse if babies are poor nappers. Lack of sleep during the day often results in an overtired baby. Overtired babies also have difficulty falling asleep at nighttime and often have more night awakenings. Some parents say their baby doesn't need daytime sleep, but this is also false. When babies miss their internal "window of opportunity" to go to sleep, they can go into a hyperalert state, which can mistakenly be interpreted as not needing much sleep. An average of 71% of babies sleep through the night at 3 months, 84% at 6 months, and 90% at 10 months of age. The babies who do sleep through the night often had a good start by being placed down for sleep when drowsy and learning to settle and fall asleep. Babies arouse naturally 4 to 6 times per night and settle back to sleep, similar to adults. We roll over or change positions and fall back into a deep sleep.

Settlers Versus Signalers

When babies wake at night, they tend to be either *settlers* or *signalers*. The settlers are only awake briefly; they may reach a light sleep state, skip the drowsy state, and then settle back into deep sleep. Then we have the signalers; they signal for mom or dad to come in and get them. They fully wake up, stay awake for a longer time, and rarely settle back to sleep on their own. When you place them down for sleep by feeding, rocking, or holding, that is how they learn to go to sleep, and they associate those rituals with sleeping. When your signaler sends out his message, watch and listen to him on a monitor but don't immediately go in to help him fall asleep. Wait to see if he can settle himself. Babies who don't know how to self-soothe wake up more fully than babies who do. This is why it is important to try to teach your baby to self-soothe during awake times, so he can do it during sleepy times. (See Chapter 3 on crying and soothing strategies.)

Sleep Associations

As previously mentioned, babies learn to associate certain conditions with going to sleep. These *sleep associations* are conditions that are present at the time of sleep onset (day or night). There are negative and positive sleep associations. *Negative* sleep associations are the primary cause of awakening during the night because the baby needs those same conditions to fall asleep. These conditions are not "negative" in and of themselves but have a negative effect on a baby's sleep because your baby cannot fall asleep without them. Negative sleep associations include feeding to sleep, being held and rocked to sleep, sleeping on a parent, massaging or rubbing their back, holding a parent's finger, or using a pacifier. Parents report that sometimes their baby falls asleep on them while they are in a recliner or on the couch; however, this is very dangerous because if the parent is tired, they may inadvertently fall asleep themselves and the baby could fall off the parent or fall in between the parent and the chair. Remember, safety is key when you are talking about sleep with babies. Sleeping in the parents' bed is a negative sleep association that is not recommended by the American Academy of Pediatrics (AAP) and is discussed in the Safe Sleep Practices section later in the chapter. Adult beds are dangerous. A parent could roll onto the baby, the baby could get suffocated in the bed linens, or the baby could even roll off the edge of the bed. Other negative sleep associations depend on movement, including riding in the car or a stroller, swinging in a baby swing, bouncing in a bouncy seat, and rocking in someone's arms. A baby may rely on just 1 or any combination of these things, but they all require a parent's presence. One mom I worked with said she had to place her baby in a stroller while she was running outside to get her to sleep, as this was the only way she could get her to sleep. This was rain or shine, hot or cold, for naps or nighttime sleep…oh my! Think of the time she spent just getting her baby to sleep!

Positive sleep associations are conditions that encourage independent sleeping. Examples are using the same crib or bassinet, the same room, and the same environment (ie, cool, dark, quiet) for sleep; using soft clothes or a sleep sack; swaddling (for younger babies); and independent sucking of a pacifier or thumb. Positive sleep associations are essential for sleep training to be successful and have a clear absence of the parent being involved. (See the Setting the Stage for Good Sleep [It Will Last a Lifetime!] section later in this chapter.)

Research has shown that there is a decrease in sudden infant death syndrome (SIDS) associated with pacifier use. (See Chapter 10 on pacifier use.) The challenge with the pacifier is that when it pops out, the baby does not have the ability to put it back in his mouth. Most babies can't put a pacifier back in their mouths themselves until they are 4 to 6 months old. At that age, I recommend you put 5 pacifiers in the crib, so your baby can successfully find one and put it in his mouth. If the pacifier does pop out while he is sleeping, wait a little before putting it back in his mouth. See if he is able to self-soothe without the pacifier. If he's still asleep, he might not need the pacifier replaced. (See the Basic Sleep Training Methods section later in this chapter).

Breastfed babies fall asleep during feeding more often than bottle-fed babies. A mom's body is warm and the baby is cradled more tightly, which can induce sleep quickly. Breastfed babies may not sleep as long (2–3 hours) as bottle-fed babies (3–5 hours) because breast (human) milk is digested more easily, and they may wake up hungry sooner. You may want to get in the habit of waking a full, breastfed baby to a drowsy state, so they can fall back to sleep on their own. Remember, feeding to sleep is a negative sleep association, so if the only way for your baby to fall asleep is by feeding, this will make it difficult for you. If you wake up your baby before placing him down in the crib, he falls asleep on his own, which is a positive sleep association. You can also breastfeed your baby earlier in your bedtime routine (eg, feed first, then change the diaper), so your baby wakes up before going to sleep.

What Is SUID?

Sudden unexpected infant death (SUID) is when an otherwise healthy infant younger than 1 year dies suddenly and unexpectedly. Included in SUID are sudden infant death syndrome (SIDS) and accidental deaths, such as accidental suffocation. Although a difficult topic to talk about, it is an important topic to bring up. About 3,700 babies in the United States die suddenly and unexpectedly each year. The highest risk period for an infant to die suddenly and unexpectedly is between 1 and 4 months of age. The best way to reduce the risk of these deaths is to follow the safe sleep practices outlined in this chapter. These include making sure that your baby is sleeping on their back on a firm, flat surface close to your bed without any bedding. Parental smoking and sleeping on the same surface as your baby increase your baby's risk of SUID, while breastfeeding decreases the risk.

It is important to know that waking to eat in the middle of the night is not necessary for your baby after 6 months of age *unless* your pediatrician has any concerns about your baby's weight. If that is the case, night feedings should continue until those concerns are resolved. We usually recommend scheduling the feedings a couple hours apart through the night rather than just letting the baby feed all night long; this is a discussion to have with your primary care physician. This way, we take advantage of your baby's normal hunger and fullness cycle, which encourages your baby to take in more calories. Babies who latch onto the breast all night long may be using the breast as a pacifier to go back to sleep rather than actually feeding for nutrition. (See Chapter 10 for more information on feeding and Chapter 11 on nutrition.)

The Importance of Sleep

Sleep professionals are beginning to understand the effect sleep has on mood, behavior, attention, and learning in adults and children. Good sleep is important for cognitive development (especially memory), and it is also important for the growth and development of the central nervous system and neural connections in the brain. Sleep allows our body and brain to rest and recover from the day's activities. The brain "cleans itself up" during sleep, especially during deep sleep. When a baby has long periods of fragmented sleep or has an inability to get into deep sleep and is sleep deprived on a regular basis, this is poor sleep. This can lead to decreased ability to focus, difficulty remembering, and difficulty calming emotions. Think of how you feel after a bad night's sleep; it's the same for babies.

Sleep challenges have a huge effect on the whole family, contributing to daytime exhaustion (both parent and baby), marital tension, and a higher risk of physical abuse. Some babies simply "grow out of" sleep problems but have more trouble getting good sleep when there are many negative sleep associations present. True chronic sleep deprivation is very rare in a young baby. Your baby may have some issues with sleep right now, but it is not considered long-term sleep deprivation. Consistently poor sleep can create an irritable baby with disorganized arousal, attention, and regulation.

Looking at Awake Times

There is a myth that a baby will go to sleep when he is tired. This is not always true, especially with fussy babies. They often go into hyperalert mode as if they are not ready for sleep. (I have heard several moms say their babies have a "fear of missing out" [FOMO]!) Looking at awake times allows for a more flexible routine than being rigid with a specific nap time every day. We try to teach parents to focus on their baby's awake times. Even if your baby only catnaps, when he wakes up, check the clock and place him down for his next sleep according to Table 9.2—but remember, fussy babies do not always give clear cues. Overtired babies often resist sleep training because they are so tired, and fussy babies often fight going to sleep. Thus, the first thing to do before sleep training is start placing your baby to sleep at regular intervals throughout the day by looking at her awake times.

Table 9.2. Awake Times by Age

Age	Length of Awake Time
1–6 wk	45 min
6–16 wk	45–80 min
4–7 mo	90–150 min

Safe Sleep Practices

The AAP has many recommendations for safe sleep. In 1996, the AAP recommended that all healthy babies be placed on their backs to sleep. As a result of this "Back to Sleep" campaign, SIDS deaths declined in the United States by about 50%. Back to sleep is the safest way for your baby to sleep, so always place your baby to sleep on her back. Always remember: "Back to sleep, tummy to play." Tummy time is important for body development, but it also helps with sleep. It strengthens the arms and coordination so a baby can move, roll around, tuck her legs, and settle into her favorite position. Eventually, babies learn to flip onto their tummies. Once your baby can flip from back to stomach and stomach to back, you do not need to keep going in and flipping her over, as it will only disrupt her sleep. Place her on her back awake and let her settle and decide what position she wants to sleep in. If your baby is a roller while she is asleep, make sure that there is nothing in her sleep area that she can get stuck against. Some babies learn to roll to their tummy, then get stuck and cry for someone to come flip them over. If this happens, practice rolling your baby from tummy to back during awake playtimes. This will help her learn this skill so she can roll herself back when she needs to.

What if My Baby Has Reflux?

Some parents worry that if their baby has reflux, she could choke if she is laid on her back for sleep. This is not true. Healthy babies without structural abnormalities like a cleft palate or a throat or windpipe disorder can be placed on their backs safely. They have a built-in mechanism in their throats that keeps them from choking. In general, it is recommended that you hold your baby with reflux upright for 20 to 30 minutes after eating. You can then put her down on her back awake when it is time to sleep. Some parents try raising the head of the crib, but usually the baby just slides down the incline to the bottom, turns to the side, or pivots all the way around so she is totally inverted, so this is not recommended. (See Chapter 2 for more information about reflux.)

Babies should always sleep on a firm, flat surface such as a mattress in a safety-approved crib or in a bassinet or a portable crib/play yard. Use a crib purchased after June 28, 2011, when a stronger safety standard became effective. Avoid cribs that have missing or broken hardware and slats that are wider than 2 3/8" apart. Avoid cutout designs in the headboard or footboard, corner posts higher than 1/16", and drop-down sides. Always have a tightly fitted sheet on the mattress, and do not surround the baby with soft objects such as blankets, pillows, stuffed animals, etc, as babies can suffocate with these objects. Bumper pads are not recommended by the AAP because babies can suffocate, get entrapped, or become strangled in the ties. Do not use a hand-me-down crib, unless you are sure it meets safety recommendations. It is also not recommended to have mobiles or hanging toys above the crib beyond 5 months of age. By this age, a baby might be mobile enough to reach up and get tangled in these toys. Babies should be lightly clothed so they don't overheat.

It is not recommended for your baby to sleep in a swing or car seat. It's OK if he falls asleep in the car seat while riding in the car, but when you arrive home, take him out of the car seat. A baby's head can droop over in these devices and block the airway, which is called *positional asphyxiation* (see Chapter 3). Your baby may also fall asleep in other baby equipment, such as a baby swing or bouncy seat; as previously stated, this presents risk for positional asphyxiation. Don't use these pieces of equipment as a sleep crutch or to help babies fall asleep. Babies should always be placed to sleep on their backs on a flat surface. If you are using these pieces of equipment and your baby falls asleep, pick him up and move him to a recommended space such as a crib or bassinet.

Inclined Sleepers and Positioners

The American Academy of Pediatrics (AAP) warns against the use of products intended for infant bed-sharing, such as baby nests, docks, pods, loungers, or nappers, because these products are not regulated and have no safety standards. The AAP also does not recommend inclined or rock-and-play sleepers, as babies can roll over in these devices and are unable to pick up their heads, which can result in suffocation or becoming trapped underneath. From January 2005 to June 2019, the Consumer Product Safety Commission (CPSC) received reports of 1,108 incidents and 73 reported deaths with these pieces of equipment. Unfortunately, some of these pieces of equipment are still being sold, so be sure to check the CPSC website (https://www.cpsc.gov) to see if any products have been deemed dangerous or recalled before purchasing them.

We know bed-sharing may be customary in some cultures and countries, but it is not recommended by the AAP. The AAP recommends that parents be separate but nearby. The policy states that babies should sleep in their parents' room until at least 6 months of age in a bassinet next to the bed. Be leery of devices that are marketed to make bed-sharing "safe"; they are not recommended. Babies can be breastfed while you are in bed but should be placed back in their bed to continue sleeping. (For more information on safe sleep, visit HealthyChildren.org.)

Sleep Challenges for Fussy Babies

Fifteen percent to 25% of parents of colicky babies report problems with sleep. Colicky babies are more unpredictable with their daytime sleep as far as how often and how long they will sleep. They are often considered cat-nappers during the day because they lack the ability to bridge light sleep to deep sleep. Unfortunately, babies who are cat-nappers are more susceptible to overstimulation. (This is the fussy baby mantra: overtired and overstimulated.)

Fussy babies also have night-to-night inconsistencies with how much they sleep and how long their stretches of sleep are. In normal sleep development, there is something called *habituation*, or the ability to tune out unimportant information. Some babies can habituate and ignore the stimuli—these babies can sleep anywhere! Fussy babies do not habituate as well. They are more affected by light and sounds during sleep and cannot tune out the external stimuli to protect their sleep. Fussy babies also tend to "shut down" when there is too much stimulation; they look like they are asleep, but often they just turn off their brains to avoid all the stimulation.

Sleep Disruptions

If your baby consistently wakes at the same time during a nap (10 or 15 minutes into the nap), she might be startling as she transitions from active sleep to quiet sleep. There are a few things you can do. Swaddling helps contain this startle so she doesn't wake up (and no swaddling if your baby is already rolling). If she wakes about the same time after being placed in the crib, another strategy you can try is to set your clock and go in a couple minutes before she starts to wake. Put your hand firmly on her chest and perhaps contain her arms; this gives her deep pressure, reduces the startle, and may help to bridge to quiet sleep. Once she is in deep sleep, you can remove your hand. If the time she awakes is inconsistent, this will not work. It also does not work if you go in after she is fully awake.

Sensitive, high-need babies may fight going to sleep frequently, but this is usually because they are overtired. They often lack the ability to self-soothe for sleep and rely on those negative associations to fall asleep, such as being fed, being held to sleep, or sleeping on the parent. Another negative association is needing movement to sleep, such as being rocked or sleeping in a swing, car seat, or stroller, which is not recommended. These types of negative associations are fine to use every once in a while to get your baby to a drowsy state but not to fall asleep. Do not make this the only way your baby can fall asleep. Some parents report they do this negative type of sleep association for sometimes up to an hour to get them to sleep, wondering if there is an easier way. Parental sleep is as high a priority as your baby's sleep, so when your baby sleeps you should sleep!

Sometimes, once colic has "resolved," sleep problems may still persist, as there are many learned behaviors or sleep associations in place. Some babies may be used to awakening more frequently. They may have fewer strategies to self-soothe, which is critical for falling asleep. It is hard to know if your baby still has colic or has a sleep problem. One way to tell is if your baby cries much less during the daytime and only at night; this may indicate a sleep issue. Sleep problems can persist into the toddler and preschool years if not addressed at a young age. It is easier to address a sleep problem in babies than in older children. More often than not, fussy babies have sleep problems with a behavioral and environmental cause. A sleep disorder is often designated for older children and usually has a medical cause. Talk with your primary care physician about the issues your baby is having with sleep; your doctor will determine if a referral to a sleep specialist is indicated.

Setting the Stage for Good Sleep (It Will Last a Lifetime!)

It is extremely important to set the stage for sleep. Go into it with appropriate expectations; know what is typical for your baby's age. A home that is noisy, has many stimulating activities, and lacks established routines—not just sleep routines but feeding and bath time routines—is not as conducive to sleep as a home with more structure, routines, and quiet and stimulating activities mixed throughout the day. It is important to ensure daily sensory experiences for your baby are not too overstimulating, especially before bedtime or nap times; this can lead to more difficulty falling asleep.

The first step is to have a sleep zone or sleep space. A *sleep zone* is where sleep occurs in the parents' room or, for older babies, the baby's room. It is ideal to take all naps and nighttime sleeps in the same place. Try not to take the baby out of her sleep zone until the morning. The room should be cool, quiet, and dark. It is recommended to use room darkening shades; they help now and in the preschool years and are typically worth the expense. Darkening the baby's sleep zone also helps the baby develop *circadian rhythms,* which are the patterns of sleep and awake that are controlled by the brain; when the baby sees light, it is time to awaken! A dim light is necessary when you need a quick diaper change, but a bright light may wake your baby up too much.

You can use sound machines (white noise) to cover environmental sounds like traffic or drown out other activities around the house. You can use it to calm and settle your baby as well. It is important to not have it too loud or too close to the baby's ear. The AAP recommends no louder than 50 decibels and at least 7 feet away from the baby. Sound machines work well; it is important that whatever sound you use should be continuous and on a loop. The device should be plugged in or fully charged so the battery doesn't die. If the sound has variations sometimes, your baby is alerted to the different sounds. As such, music or lullabies are not the best choice. You can incorporate these into your sleep routine, but they are not ideal for sleeping. Some popular sounds are those of a fan, static, or a humidifier, as they are constant and not variable. A babbling brook may sound nice but could be too alerting because there is variability in its sounds. You can easily wean your baby off the sound machine by turning the volume down, and then turning it off completely when you have sleep trained your baby successfully.

Sleep Clothing

What your baby sleeps in is also part of setting the stage for sleep. There are many sleep sacks on the market that are very useful. They keep babies warm and snug, giving babies a sense of security. Be aware that some sleep sacks keep the baby too restrained and do not allow the baby to get her hand to her mouth or to roll to her side, both self-soothing strategies. (Remember, no blankets in the crib; a sleep sack will do the job.) It may be fun to dress up your baby in those cute outfits with flowers or decorations, but they are not ideal for sleeping. When you are around the house, keep your baby in onesies or comfortable clothes to sleep in, so you don't have to keep changing her clothes. Swaddling is also a great option for the younger baby (see Chapter 12). Research shows swaddled infants wake less often. Swaddling is used to induce sleep and reduce crying with fussy babies. (Remember, once your baby starts rolling you need to take her out of the swaddle.)

A Sleep Routine

Another important thing when setting the stage is to have a routine. You can start early with a routine, and it is never too late to implement, but it is best to have the routine somewhat in place by 3 months of age. Your routine should be somewhat flexible depending on your baby's hunger cues. Often younger babies' schedules do not allow for a strict routine because they sleep more frequently than eat, which as long as you are reading your baby, is totally fine. Soothing interactions to prepare for sleep can involve a wide variety of actions, including a bath, a massage, reading a story, reciting prayers, or singing a song. Massage has been proven to help with sleep. Be aware that sometimes baths or massages may be too alerting, so read your baby's cues. If a bath or a massage gets them too excited, then try it at another time of day, not before bed. If you want to feed during the routine, that is OK, but remember, we want your baby to be drowsy, not sound asleep, which often happens if you feed your baby just prior to sleep. If you want to get out of the nursing-to-sleep habit, move the feeding earlier in the routine. Routines should take 15 to 20 minutes (a little longer if you incorporate a bath or a massage), but they should be no more than 30 minutes. For naps, you can follow the same routine but make it shorter. As you have learned there are a lot of components to setting the stage for good sleep. If you have not started a routine, now is the time! Don't feel overwhelmed, just do a little at a time and soon you will have an ideal "sleep zone."

What Is Sleep Training and Is It for You?

Sleep training involves teaching your baby to fall asleep and return to sleep on his own when he awakens in the middle of the night. Some babies do not have to be sleep trained; they just happen to have the ability to fall asleep naturally, without any negative sleep associations. However, fussy or high-need babies usually need some sort of sleep training, often because several negative sleep associations may already be in place. Sleep experts recommend sleep training should be done when your baby is 4 months or older. By this time, there is usually a pattern with his sleep-wake cycles, and he may be able to self-soothe. There is no one-size-fits-all approach when it comes to sleep training, and there is no right or wrong way to sleep train. It is a family decision and it depends on your parenting style, your tolerance for your baby's crying, and your baby's temperament. People (including your parents, in-laws, or friends) often have strong opinions about the right way to sleep train. Remember to be confident in your choice and stick with it!

The sleep behaviors to target with sleep training include

- Going to sleep while drowsy
- Falling asleep on his own
- Staying asleep
- Reaching a quiet state of sleep
- Falling back to sleep when awakened

If these are not the behaviors you aim to achieve, now may not be the time to start sleep training. The most important thing you can do as parents is to understand what sleep training is, figure out if you are ready to attempt it, and understand the different approaches that are used. There are several tips to follow while deciding whether to sleep train.

- Review the methods of sleep training and decide together which method fits with your family the best.
- Be absolutely consistent once you decide to sleep train. Babies are very smart; if you do well for 3 days with the routine of sleep training and then throw in the towel, what has your baby learned? That you will eventually give in. Be consistent and don't give up!
- Make sure you are emotionally ready to sleep train and that you have the confidence to follow through. If you have any doubt, you are not ready to sleep train. Some babies are very easy to sleep train and some take more work, so you have to be patient and ready emotionally if your baby takes a little longer.
- Pick an ideal time to start sleep training. Don't start the sleep training if you have vacations planned or if there is going to be a disruption to your normal life, such as overnight visitors or a parent out of town for longer than is typical. If you or your baby has an upcoming medical procedure scheduled, wait until after it is done and you or your baby has recovered comfortably. How long sleep training takes varies, but make sure to free your schedule for about 2 weeks just in case.

If you have addressed these tips, you are ready to sleep train! When starting, make sure to give your baby extra attention during the day so she feels loved and responded to. There are 3 basic methods of sleep training and variations in all of them, depending on the source. There are many books dedicated specifically to sleep for all ages that include recommendations for sleep training. Following is a brief overview of each approach to help you understand the basics and start the process. This brief overview is focused on babies 6 months and younger. It is important to know that all these methods work. Babies do cry during sleep training; there isn't really a no-cry way to sleep train. The methods vary in duration or length of training because every baby and every set of parents is different. In all these methods, *the first thing to remember is to place your baby down drowsy, not asleep.*

Basic Sleep Training Methods

Cry It Out Method (or Standard Extinction)

This approach sometimes gets a bad rap, as some may feel you are "abandoning" your baby and not listening to her concerns. There are no studies that prove that the cry it out method has any adverse effect on parent-baby attachment or the emotional development of the baby.

Make sure your baby is changed, well fed, and ready for sleep (remember to look at her awake time!). Place your baby in the crib drowsy but awake and leave the room, making the goodbye short and sweet. Let her cry until she falls asleep on her own. If she wakes up, check on her on the monitor, not in person. Let her cry until she goes back to sleep. The crib can be in your room if your baby is younger than 6 months, but be very quiet when you turn in for the night. If your baby wakes up, do not attend to her. Allow her to self-soothe herself back to sleep. This method has been around for years, is the most well-known approach, and is often recommended by family, friends, and even some pediatricians. It can be tough on parents who cannot bear to hear their baby cry. If that is you, you may want to try one of the other approaches.

Continue this method for every nap and overnight sleep until your baby is consistently going to sleep on her own.

Checking In (Ferber) Method

Place your baby in her crib drowsy but awake. Make your goodbye short and sweet and leave. The idea is that you check in every 5 minutes and continue check-ins every 5 minutes if your baby is still crying. Some people increase the increments of time throughout the night; for example, the first check-in is within 5 minutes, the second is within 7 minutes, the third is within 9 minutes, and so on. You can also change the increments of time each night; for example, the first night is 5 minutes for every awakening, the second night is 7 minutes, the third night is 9 minutes, and so on. How you approach it is totally up to you; just decide ahead of time what your plan is so both parents can implement it accurately and stay consistent.

During your first or initial check-in, if your baby is still crying, reassure her that she is OK but don't pick her up. Make sure check-ins are brief with no emotion. You can replace a pacifier if needed, but don't stay in the room longer than 30 seconds.

Continue this process every 5 minutes (or your decided time) until she falls asleep. If she wakes up, go back to checking every 5 minutes (or your decided time).

Maintain this for every nap and overnight sleep until your baby is consistently going to sleep on her own.

Gradual Extinction (Also Known as Sleep Coaching or Fading Adult Intervention)

In this approach, place your baby in his crib drowsy but awake and then stand next to the crib. He can see you, hear you, and feel you (3 sensory systems of vision, hearing, and touch). You can talk to him, shush him, and rub his back; just don't pick him up and hold him. Do this until he falls asleep on his own, and then leave the room. If he wakes up, go back in, but don't pick him up. Stand with him and repeat the same strategies as before.

The next night, eliminate one of the sensations. He can always see you, so plan for that to be the last sensation to drop. You can either talk to him or rub his back but not both. You can tailor this step as needed; for example, you can use all the sensations for a week and then change a sensation, rather than changing something every night. If your baby wakes up, go back in, but don't pick him up. Stand next to the crib and repeat the same strategies as before.

The next night, remove the other sensation; he can see you, but don't do anything else. Simply stand next to the crib without engaging with him. This can be the hardest night! If he wakes up, go back in, don't pick him up, and just stand next to him. This approach is very hard to do if you are the kind of parent who can't stand it when your baby cries, as you cannot do anything on this night using this approach. That is why you need to familiarize yourself with all the approaches and see which one fits best with your family.

Continue this for every nap and overnight sleep until your baby is consistently going to sleep on his own. On the final night, stand halfway between the crib and the door, so he can still see you, but he is totally settling on his own.

Bottom Line

Pick what works for you and be consistent! Some parents inadvertently use a combination of the sleep training approaches, but this can seem confusing to your baby. "How come sometimes I have to cry for a long time and sometimes it is only 5 minutes?" Be consistent with the type of training you decide on. Sometimes babies get very upset and vomit, or they may have a poopy diaper. In these cases, clean them up, change their diaper, and place them back in the crib to continue with the sleep training method you have been doing. It is best if you sleep train for naps and nighttime sleep at the same time. I always recommend starting the sleep training at bedtime first. You can sleep train for nighttime first and then for naps, but it will take longer for both to be well-established, so it is best to sleep train at the same time.

You can still sleep train if your baby awakens for nighttime feedings; it's just a little trickier! Remember, a typical 6-month-old does not have to wake for nighttime feedings. If your baby has a medical reason she still has to eat in the middle of the night, you can still sleep train and schedule the feeding. When it is time to eat, you wake your baby. When she wakes up on her own, she needs to fall back to sleep. Essentially, your baby will learn that when you wake her, she gets fed, but when she wakes up, she needs to fall back to sleep. It may seem odd to have to wake a baby up, but it communicates the right message to her.

It would be great if you only had to sleep train your baby once; however, that is not always the case. Vacations, illnesses, life transitions such as moving or a parent returning to work, time changes, etc, can disrupt your baby's sleep pattern. Teething is also a big challenge; don't wait until teething is over to sleep train because your baby will be teething for several years until all the baby teeth come in. If you have to sleep train your baby again after one of these situations, it is usually much easier the second time around. There may also be "sleep regression"—sometimes everything is going well, and then all of a sudden, your baby starts waking again. Research disputes that sleep regressions happen at a set time or month during your baby's life. They usually happen when there are some developmental changes, such as learning how to get into a sitting position or pulling to stand, or cognitive gains, such as object permanence or separation anxiety. Try to stick with the sleep training method you used the first time when she was successfully sleep trained; it will be easier this time for both of you. When life gets in the way and you get off track, start back up again when things settle down.

Sleep is a valuable commodity for everyone in the family! Hopefully, these sleep strategies gave you some insight into the importance of sleep and helped you understand why fussy babies struggle. Now that you have learned how to have a good, safe sleep environment, how to sleep train your baby, and how to establish good sleep routines, everyone will have better sleep!

> "I am so glad I learned about sleep training. My husband and I made a decision to use the checking-in method. He came home from work the first night we were going to attempt it and asked if I gave up. I said no, the twins are sleeping and fell asleep on their own! It made such a difference to everyone; I wish I would have tried it sooner!"
>
> Mother of 8-month-old twins

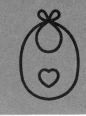

Chapter 10

Feeding Challenges and the Fussy Baby

Parents often anticipate that feeding their baby will be a warm, bonding experience. No one can fully prepare a parent for the stress and worry of having a baby who is challenging to feed. Why would a baby not eat? Why would she push the bottle away and stop eating after only 1 or 2 ounces when she must still be hungry? When she is not gaining enough weight and your pediatrician tells you to "feed your baby more," it's even more upsetting when she *won't*. Luckily, there are tools and tips that can help.

> ### Did You Know?
> Feeding challenges can occur in 25% to 36% of fussy babies.

To help your baby feed better, it is important to first find out if the feeding challenges are solely related to colic or fussiness, or if there could be underlying swallowing difficulty (a disorder called *dysphagia*). The discomfort of a swallowing disorder can make fussiness worse. If your baby is fussy only during feeding times, a thorough medical evaluation may help rule out a swallowing disorder. Risk of having a swallowing disorder is higher in babies with a history of other medical problems, such as preterm birth, breathing issues, or differences in structures of the face or mouth. A pediatric speech-language pathologist who specializes in swallowing can help assess if your baby has symptoms of a swallowing disorder.

Typical Feeding and Swallowing Patterns

Swallowing is one of the most complex processes of the body. It's amazing that something that requires coordination of so many systems, muscles, and nerves simply happens for most of us, hundreds of times a day, without even thinking about it.

Success with feeding can depend on a variety of factors, such as your baby's ability to stay calm to complete his feed, the positioning of his head and neck, the flow of the nipple, and sucking skills. A baby shows he's hungry with cues such as *rooting*. Rooting is when a touch to the lips or cheeks makes your baby turn his head with his mouth open toward the breast or bottle. Once the nipple is in his mouth, he quickly begins a strong, rhythmic sucking pattern: suck, swallow, breathe. This cycle occurs continuously, and the pattern of sucking appears organized, with rhythmical bursts of sucking and breathing.

If you listen carefully during a feeding, you can hear the exhale after each swallow. Every so often, he may pause after several cycles to take a few additional catch-up breaths. Breathing and swallowing are so finely coordinated that coughing, choking, or gagging hardly ever happens.

When a baby struggles to feed, this may involve a lack of rooting, poor sucking, and longer than normal feedings. Babies with colic often struggle with organizing the process of feeding. They may not be able to organize and coordinate the important suck, swallow, breathe pattern. A disorganized suck pattern with no rhythm may occur; there may be no predictable pauses, and suck bursts may be too short or too long. This affects the length of the feeding and the timing of the coordination between breathing and swallowing. Gagging, coughing, choking events may occur if the coordination is impaired.

The 3 Phases of Swallowing

There are 3 primary phases of swallowing: *oral phase, pharyngeal phase,* and *esophageal phase.*

Oral Phase

This phase involves the structures and muscles of the mouth, including the lips, cheeks, and tongue. A newborn has early reflexes of rooting and sucking. She also has fat pads in her cheeks, which allows her to latch with a strong seal around a nipple.

Rooting and sucking are reflexive during the first 2 months after birth. Between 2 and 4 months they become voluntary and a baby develops control to stop or start sucking. It also allows her to refuse to suck on a breast or bottle and push out the nipple with her tongue.

Pharyngeal Phase

The pharyngeal phase is involuntary, a reflex controlled by the brain. It is triggered once food or liquid passes into the throat, or *pharynx*. Below the throat are 2 parallel pipes. The windpipe, or trachea, is in front of the *esophagus*. The trachea is for breathing and the esophagus is the food pipe that connects to the stomach. Have you noticed that it is impossible to breathe and swallow at the same time? The windpipe has a type of doorway that is open during breathing but closes during swallowing, so food passes through the throat and down into the esophagus and not down the windpipe. If food enters the trachea, it is termed *aspiration* (commonly referred to as something going down "the wrong pipe"), which leads to choking or coughing. Along with the reflexes, the anatomy of the throat begins to change between 2 and 4 months of age as a baby grows. The neck becomes longer, moving the structures farther apart, and that requires swallowing to perform more precisely. Dysphagia may be present at birth, but feeding or swallowing problems can also begin at about this time, as the growth and changes in the mouth and throat take place.

Did You Know?

Up to 3% of the population is born with a *tongue-tie*, which is also known as a tight lingual frenulum or ankyloglossia. Releasing a tongue-tie does not always improve nursing issues. If a tongue-tie is present, a lactation consultation should always be done first to make sure latch and positioning are appropriate. If a mother continues to feel pain with nursing and/or a poor latch after she receives support from a lactation consultant, she should discuss this with her primary care physician. The physician may refer the baby to see either an ear, nose, and throat specialist or a pediatric dentist. These specialists can determine not only the presence of a tongue-tie but its effect on the tongue function.

Esophageal Phase

This is also an involuntary phase. Food passes through the esophagus and is emptied into the stomach. If there are problems with this part of the process, they are usually taken care of by a *gastroenterologist* (a doctor who specializes in the stomach and lower parts of the digestive system).

Dysphagia: Signs and Symptoms

Dysphagia can occur in any or all of the phases of swallowing. It may be caused by disorganized feeding skills; poor coordination of the suck, swallow, breathe pattern; or an immature nervous system. Table 10.1 reviews symptoms of oral versus pharyngeal dysphagia.

Table 10.1. Oral and Pharyngeal Dysphagia

Oral Dysphagia	Pharyngeal Dysphagia
Baby attempts to latch to a pacifier but gags or is unable to suck on a pacifier	Delayed swallow
Short sucking bursts, frequent pauses	Loud/hard swallows
Weak or disorganized suck	Choking
Pulling off or biting the nipple	Coughing
Gagging on the nipple	Congestion during/after feeding
Spilling/spitting milk	Red/watery eyes
Pooling milk in the mouth	Color changes to the face or lips

Difficulty in the pharyngeal phase of swallowing is more concerning, as it can lead to poor weight gain as well as respiratory illnesses. A primary concern when these characteristics are present is *aspiration*. Aspiration means the food has traveled down the trachea and passed into the lungs. An occasional cough during feeding is considered acceptable, but if the coughing with feeding occurs frequently over time it may become a serious medical problem. It is concerning if a baby coughs during every feeding or multiple times in a feeding.

Aspiration may lead to colds, congestion, or, eventually, pneumonia. It is even more dangerous when the aspiration is "silent." *Silent aspiration* is when the food goes down the wrong pipe without the baby coughing. As many as

95% of babies who aspirate have episodes of silent aspiration. They may be choking without any coughing. In these cases, watch for subtle symptoms such as increased congestion during or after a feeding and red or watery eyes while eating. Another major red flag is aversive behaviors to eating, including feeding refusals. It is important to watch out for these symptoms if a baby also has weight loss or poor weight gain. If you notice these symptoms, your primary care physician may recommend a formal swallow test. A consultation with a speech-language pathologist may help to confirm the need for a swallow test or suggest modifications to help your baby feed safely and efficiently. There are 2 types of swallow tests that can be performed. These tests can show if your baby has dysphagia and is aspirating. They can also determine what strategies can help reduce this risk and assist a baby in eating safely.

- **Fiberoptic endoscopic swallow study.** A tube with a tiny camera is inserted through the nose and into the throat by an ear, nose, and throat specialist while the speech-language pathologist evaluates the swallow.
- **Video fluoroscopic swallow study.** A baby drinks barium during an x-ray of the throat while a speech-language pathologist and radiologist evaluate the swallow.

Feeding Challenges and the Fussy Baby

Colic and fussiness can make feeding difficult—no argument here! Symptoms of a swallowing disorder can overlap with those of poor state regulation (ie, the disorganized feeding ability), so it can be hard to tell one from the other. The disorganized feeder shows problems with sucking for continuous cycles, staying alert enough to complete a full feed, and giving cues for being ready to eat. Table 10.2 outlines common symptoms. Keep in mind that any given baby may not have all the possible symptoms.

Your baby communicates with her behavior when something is not going well or she needs more support during a feeding. The behaviors we look for are referred to as *signs or symptoms of distress*. As you identify the signs of distress you can respond with a strategy. Common signs of distress during the feeding include

- Arching
- Head turning
- Facial grimace
- Splaying out of the fingers
- Eyebrow raising
- Hard eye close
- Extraneous movements or fidgeting with hands/feet
- Crying
- Shutting down/falling asleep

Table 10.2. Symptoms of Disorganized Bottle-feeding or Breastfeeding

Body is squirmy and active
Gagging with presentation of the nipple
Spillage when distracted
Unable to re-latch if interrupted
Prefers to feed when asleep or very drowsy (also called "dream feeding")
Pulling on/off the nipple
Easily distracted
Short sucking bursts
Crying, batting, or pushing the nipple away
Unable to calm enough to eat
Takes more than 30 minutes to feed
Can only be fed by 1 person or in 1 room
Air swallowing, gulping
Fidgeting with hands/feet during feeding
Very busy when nursing, playing excessively with your shirt, hair, hand, jewelry
Head turning while sucking

It is important to be aware that a baby's signs of stress mean just that: stress. The only way she has to communicate is through her behavior, because she cannot explain it to you! People have often associated a baby's stress sign of arching the body with acid reflux, but arching behavior during or before a feeding is not specific to reflux; it's simply a sign of stress. We have to work out what the signs may mean in the context in which we see them. If they happen during the feeding, we can analyze what is not working about that particular feed and figure out strategies to help.

Feeding Strategies

If you and your baby truly struggle with feedings, it is important to work with a qualified specialist. A medical professional should always guide interventions such as changing formulas, thickening liquids, or adding medications. If done incorrectly, these changes can make feedings even more difficult, cause your baby to avoid feeding, or even lead to dehydration or other harm.

The following strategies may be useful before or during a feeding for a baby with poor state regulation, who can't organize his feeding functions. Remember, there is no one-size-fits-all solution. The best advice: be *predictable*. Even if your baby is unpredictable or inconsistent with feedings, he can learn from your consistencies and avoidance of too much change. If your baby struggles to eat to the point that you feel that you need to force-feed, please seek guidance. Force-feeding, even if it's gentle, can cause a baby to develop an oral aversion.

Predictable Routines

Before you work on feeding techniques, establish a predictable environment and routine. A baby with poor state regulation will benefit from feeding associations. Similar to sleep associations, they cue the baby that it's time to eat. Daily life may not always allow you to keep these routines, but try to feed your baby in the same place as much as you can. In this room, limit noise and distractions such as television. Soothing sounds, such as a fan or soft music, are OK. Think about which way your baby will face. Is the baby distracted by looking out the window or an open door? Some babies like a dimly lit room so they can focus their attention on eating. Siblings can be distracting too, so this may be a good opportunity for your partner or another family member to set aside special activities just for them during baby's feeding time. Keep everything you need handy and ready to go before you feed your baby. A fussy baby is easily distracted by interruptions. Sometimes these interruptions end the feeding too early, before the baby has eaten enough. You don't want to have to pause the feeding to grab a burp cloth! If bottle-feeding, it may also be helpful to prepare the bottle with a little extra formula or expressed breast milk if you can spare it in case your baby wants to eat more. Pausing to refill the bottle is another interruption that could end the feed.

If your routine is to feed after your baby wakes, watch out for those transitions! While some babies tolerate clothing changes, diaper changes, and transitioning from their bassinet or crib to another room, others become overstimulated and are then unable to calm to eat well. If this is the case, adjust your routine to fit your baby's needs. It's OK to feed first and then change an outfit or diaper if that's what works better for now.

The Feeders

Be thoughtful about how many people are involved in feeding your baby. Feeding is a relationship you work on with your baby, so try to limit the number of others who feed her as much as possible. This may mean it's just you and your partner. This can be very difficult for well-intentioned family members and friends. Remind them that you are working on predictable feedings. Everyone has a slightly different "style" in how they position or how much they focus or understand a baby's cues. Changes in a feeding routine may confuse your baby, and she may feel as if she is starting all over again!

If your baby attends child care, talk to the providers about choosing a primary feeder. Let them know what is going on with your baby's needs, and they will likely be able to accommodate your routines. Once your baby starts to show she understands your feeding routines and accepts the bottle more easily, you can then try to expand the number of people that offer her feedings.

Feeding Schedule

Stick to a schedule that complements your baby's states. Some babies need to really feel hunger and benefit from longer stretches rather than more frequent feeds (eg, give 3 ounces every 3 to 4 hours rather than 1 to 2 ounces every 1 to 2 hours). This may contradict "old school" advice to feed your baby more frequently with small volumes. However, babies with poor state regulation often eat better with a longer stretch between feeds instead of grazing on small volumes. The small volumes sometimes can fill your baby up enough to take the edge off his hunger, and he may refuse more. This can be especially common if he learns you will feed him multiple times within the hour or an hour later. Ask your baby's pediatrician how long your baby can go between feedings. Try to set a schedule, with some flexibility. For example, your baby may eat every 3 to 3½ hours. Instead of offering a feeding to your baby exactly at the 3-hour mark, try to watch for hunger cues.

When it is getting near feeding time on the schedule you set, watch for subtle cues that your baby is hungry, such as mouthing on his hands, excitement when he sees the bottle, or vigorous sucking on a pacifier. Crying is not the only hunger cue, so avoid waiting until your baby is crying inconsolably, as he may not be able to calm himself enough to focus on feeding. A baby feeds best when in a quiet, calm state at the start of the feed.

If you breastfeed your baby, you may notice he nurses for nourishment and for comfort too. Establishing a feeding schedule can be extremely challenging in this case but may be a goal if your baby struggles to eat. If you prefer to focus on working out a routine for nursing or want to reduce comfort nursing, it may be useful to have a support system. This may include your partner and a lactation consultant. Your partner can take a turn to try to help your baby soothe after he had a good meal. A lactation consultant can also help you figure out your baby's transfer skills and intake during a nursing session to help you feel confident that your baby is eating enough. Once you have a good understanding of your baby's skills, it will be easier to identify hunger cues by thinking about the last time your baby fed. For example, how long did the feeding last? Did he empty the breast when he ate? Let your lactation consultant know what your goals are so the consultant can assist accordingly.

Bottle Options

If you bottle-feed, stop trying new bottles! Every time your baby is introduced to a new bottle, she has to adapt her sucking pattern for that bottle (the same goes for pacifiers). There is no "magical" bottle. Bottle shapes, nipple sizes, and flows vary a lot among brands. For example, a wide-based nipple tends to flow faster than a narrow-based one. Manufacturers offer suggested flows based on age, but there is wide variability. A brand may advertise its bottle nipple as a "slow flow," but it might flow faster than a "slow flow" nipple of another brand. When a baby can't keep up with the flow of a nipple, she will spit out the milk, let it leak from the sides of her mouth, or sound like she is gulping when she swallows. This causes a baby to become more disorganized as she tries to cope, often leading to more fussiness with a feed. Therefore, a slower-flow nipple may be more effective. It is challenging to know which brand will be best for your baby; there are charts and studies that compare nipple flow rates, but they should be used only as guides. They are not "exacts" because the flow is also affected by the strength of your baby's suck and the anatomy of your baby's mouth.

If you've tried many bottles already, pick one with which you know your baby has had at least 1 good feeding or that you use most often. Make sure to check the flow rate. Most brands have different-sized nipples. Brands will label their flow rates by rate, age, or a number. Rate is usually classified as "preemie, slow, medium, fast." Some bottle brands also have "Y" cut nipples, which should not be used, as they are extremely fast flowing and will cause a young baby to choke. Number labels are "0, 1, 2, 3," and age ranges are typically "newborn, 0–3 months, 3–6 month, 6–9 months." If a flow rate is too fast, it's OK to try a slower flow or stick to the same flow even if your baby is past the indicated age labeled on the nipple. If a baby doesn't graduate to a faster flow, it doesn't mean that there is something wrong with him. There is no "reward" for moving up a nipple size! The nipple size should be selected based on your baby's sucking strength and swallowing coordination.

Positioning

Choose a chair where you can comfortably hold your baby. Chairs with armrests help you support and contain your baby close to your body. Some babies even enjoy being swaddled during a feed. When holding your baby for feeding, pay attention to the position of your baby's head and hands.

First, check the head and neck positioning. It is best to have good alignment of the head, neck, and trunk. If you look in the mirror while holding your baby in this position, you will see that you can draw an imaginary straight line starting from the ears and down to the shoulders and the hips (Figure 10.1). The head will not be extended back or tucked too close to the body. Neither of those are comfortable for baby to swallow!

One mom I worked with experienced back problems and was just not able to be comfortable while attempting to align her baby's head and neck with her body. Her baby continued to turn her head to the side and arch, causing mom discomfort when she leaned forward to readjust her baby. She found using a nursing pillow on her lap really helped. Her baby's body was fully supported, and the pillow freed her to use her hands to concentrate on supporting the head and neck.

Next, check where your baby holds his hands. You may notice your baby either clasps his hands or keeps them near each other, close to his chest or chin when he is feeding best. Both of these positions are important, as they support the natural organization and coordination of sucking and swallowing. If a baby is disorganized, his arms may be held out, away from his body or down at his sides. Sometimes this also changes the head position, and you may notice your baby's head extend back instead of staying in the neutral aligned position that is preferred (Figure 10.2). These positions can affect the strength of the suck and the coordination of the suck, swallow, breathe pattern. Think about what happens to your tongue when your head is tilted

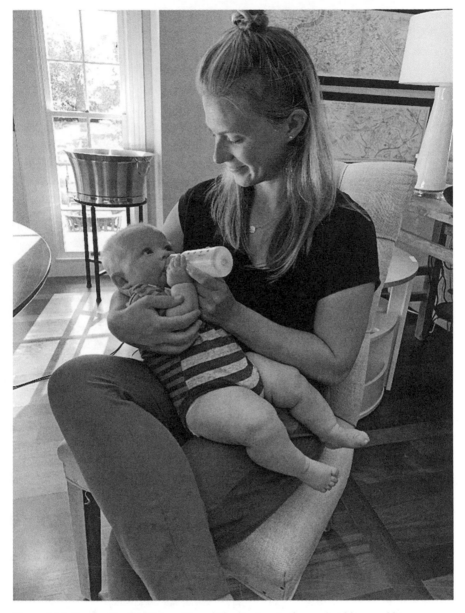

Figure 10.1. Supportive feeding position with alignment of ears, shoulders, and hips.

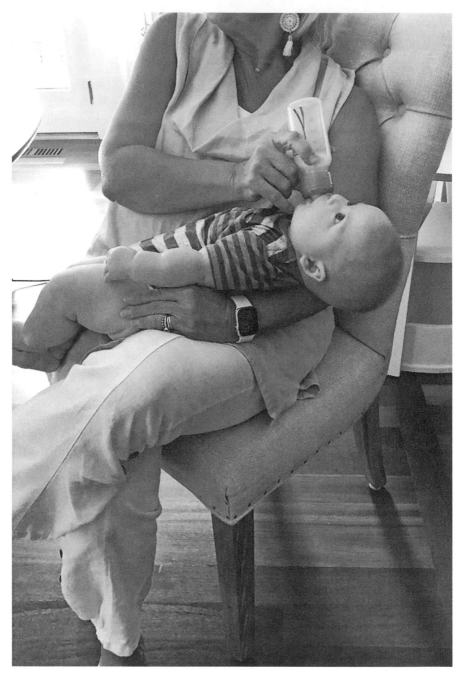

Figure 10.2. Unsupported feeding position. Baby's head is hyperextended and arms are down at the sides.

back; your tongue may retract and fall away from the roof of your mouth. A baby uses his tongue to strip a nipple and extract milk, so we want to make sure the seal and latch are strong and avoid tongue retraction. Tilting the head back can also affect swallowing. When you tilt your head back to swallow, liquid may travel even faster due to gravity. If it travels too fast, a baby can swallow air or choke. If your baby struggles to maintain his hands and head in the flexed and midline position, a swaddle can be handy. Be careful not to swaddle with his arms down, though, as they should be in the middle of the body to avoid his head tilting back.

For some parents, alternative positions will do the trick. One baby had been identified with dysphagia and required alterations to her feeding position to eat. Because feeding had been causing discomfort, she was defensive to eating. This baby fed best when reclined in a supportive nursing pillow. Mom and dad used extra blankets to support her bottom so she wouldn't slide down. This position worked wonderfully for this family because they could easily see her face and body as they watched her cues. Just remember, if you choose to feed your baby while she is not being held in your arms, you must always supervise her for safety!

Organize the Mouth

During mouthing, a baby brings her hands to her mouth or roots for a pacifier or nipple to indicate hunger. This can be very organizing for your baby's mouth and prepares her to feed. Help your baby to organize her mouth by offering a favorite pacifier or assisting her to bring her hands to her mouth.

Pacifier use can be very helpful during this stage in development with a fussy baby. The pacifier can help her self-regulate, calm, and even prepare her mouth for the feed. Think of the pacifier as stretching before a workout. There are many options for pacifiers. Just like the bottle, use what works. If your baby has had trouble sustaining sucking with the pacifier but still shows interest, try a pacifier that has a shorter or flatter-shaped nipple and has a butterfly-shaped guard that curves to the face. These are less likely to fall out. If the pacifier is more frustrating than helpful but your baby really wants nonnutritive sucking, help her hold it in place for now or allow your baby to suckle on a clean finger. Sucking is a reflex up to 4 months of age, and babies will readily accept a stimulus that works for their level of coordination. If they refuse, it most likely is because of swallowing or feeding issues rather than the pacifier itself.

Some caregivers worry that a pacifier may harm a baby's teeth, be too difficult to wean, or work against nursing due to nipple confusion. Most babies at this young age can easily transition between nutritive (feeding at breast or bottle) and nonnutritive (pacifier) sucking. In addition, most babies younger than 6 months do not have teeth yet, or the dentition is just starting to emerge. So, if a pacifier helps your baby calm, use it to help her *now*, without any worries.

Bottle-feeding Techniques

Once you are ready to offer a bottle, do so slowly. To help your baby latch, place the nipple at your baby's lips and allow him to open his mouth to show you he is ready. Keep the bottle slightly tipped downward so there is no milk in the nipple; you can easily glide it in along the roof of his mouth without touching the tongue or dripping milk (Figure 10.3). If a bottle drips milk in your baby's mouth before he is ready, it can surprise him and cause him to gag (Figure 10.4). Presenting the nipple empty in this way helps to avoid dripping until he is ready to start sucking and swallowing.

If your baby turns his head away, do not "chase" him with the bottle. He knows where it is and will turn his head back to greet the nipple when he is ready. If he becomes upset to the point of crying, try to calm him by placing the bottle out of sight and offering a pacifier or "shushing" sound. If you can, avoid excessive bouncing or fast rocking, as this may stimulate your baby too much for feeding.

Once your baby has latched, watch for his cues. If he is comfortable, you will not notice much! He may keep his hands in the middle, running his fingers along his shirt. He might look up at you or stare at the fan in the room. However, during active sucking or swallowing, you may also notice your baby showing some stress cues. He may turn his head sharply away from the nipple, push out the nipple with his tongue and gag, or spill milk out the sides of his mouth. Stress cues can be seen on his face with facial grimaces, high eyebrow raises, hard eye closing, and hands splaying and batting away at the bottle. If this happens, help your baby to feel in control with pacing.

Pacing is a technique that allows your baby to catch up on breathing or swallowing by imposing a break, and it can be done without fully removing the bottle from her mouth. If you start to notice your baby is showing a stress cue, pace her before the stress cues become so evident that she is trying to escape the bottle. Some of these early cues might be the milk slightly pooling at the corner of her lips, her swallows getting louder, or a

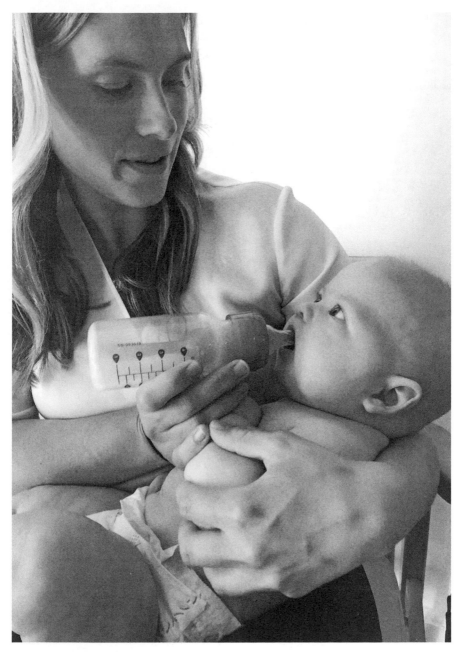

Figure 10.3. Nipple presented empty.

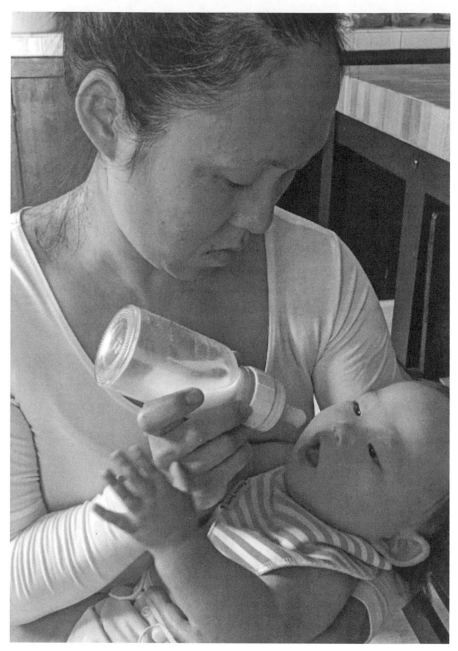

Figure 10.4. Nipple presented full, dripping.

worried look on her face. If you notice these, simply tip the bottle down so that the milk empties from the nipple (Figure 10.5). She may continue to suck a couple of times before she realizes what you are doing. Do not worry about her swallowing too much air when you practice this. It is better to not completely remove the bottle from her mouth because interruptions may be too disrupting. She will get the hang of it and start to understand that this is a break. She may even start to pause and take breaks on her own after a few tries! This break should last only for a couple of seconds, just long enough to take some catch-up breaths and swallow whatever remains in her mouth. She will let you know she is ready for more when she starts sucking again. That's when you tilt the bottle back up so the nipple refills with milk.

If she pulls her mouth off the nipple or turns her head sharply away from the bottle, allow her to turn her head away and back to the nipple when she is ready for more. Keeping the nipple empty during these more evident stress cues also prevents unexpected dripping of milk.

This pacing technique can be used any time during the feeding. Some babies need it more often in the beginning of a feed, when they are sucking vigorously, but do not need help once they are in a good rhythm. Other babies may need some help to coordinate their suck, swallow, breathe pattern for most of the feeding until they gain some more feeding experience. However, if you feel your baby needs an excessive amount of pacing with almost every suck or every couple of sucks, it likely means that the flow is still too fast, or she may need to see a feeding specialist to work on her coordination.

If your baby becomes upset to the point of crying and is no longer calm enough to feed, take a true rest break. Give her some floor time or use other calming strategies without the bottle in sight. She may take her pacifier again, which is a nice, organizing task associated with the feeding. Your baby may take a few rest breaks during a feeding as needed. Once she is calmed, it will be easier to start again with slow reintroduction of the empty nipple.

Even if she does not consistently accept the nipple when it is time to feed, be consistent in how you respond with your strategies of presenting the nipple empty, using the appropriate nipple flow rate, pacing, and rest breaks so she knows what to expect. Never pressure your baby by forcing her to keep sucking when she needs a break or when she is not ready. Trying the bottle over and over again after it's been longer than 30 minutes can also make eating feel like a chore for both you and your baby, so it's important to also consider a time limit.

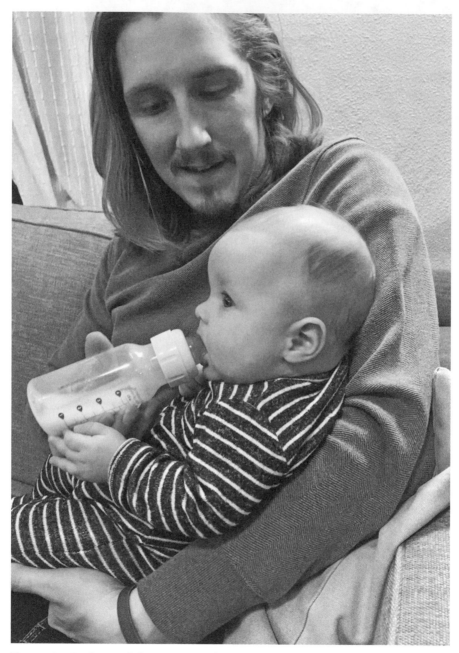

Figure 10.5. Bottle tipped down to empty the nipple during pacing.

Length of the Feeding

It is recommended to keep feedings to 30 minutes or less. Your baby's swallowing skills may become fatigued if the feed is longer than 30 minutes, causing more disorganization. When a baby becomes increasingly disorganized from fatigue, you will see continuously shorter suck bursts and frequent pauses, resulting in longer feeding times of just a small amount. Remember, the suck, swallow, breathe process is an aerobic activity for your baby. This is part of why it is not recommended to bottle-feed beyond 30 minutes.

If your baby took a small but acceptable amount within this time frame, it's OK to stop the feed and wait until the next scheduled time to offer more. Trying for another hour to get an extra ounce fed may help in the short term but will not help for your long-term goals of consistent, calm feeding. It creates more stress for you and your baby and can lead your baby to feel he is being forced to eat. If your baby is taking a dangerously low volume over a 24-hour period, contact your primary care physician immediately. Your doctor can provide you with guidance about acceptable amounts of feeding and help ease your stress during this learning period.

Burping

As your baby feeds, avoid interrupting to burp her unless she initiates a break. Burping can be offered if she begins to disengage and shows discomfort from swallowing air. You can also offer it at the very end of the feeding. Air swallowing can occur for multiple reasons. If you notice that your baby collapses the nipple during feeding, she may benefit from a vented bottle system to eliminate this problem. If you make formula and notice that shaking the mix causes a lot of air bubbles, try stirring it or making it ahead of time so the bubbles have time to settle. Most formula containers provide instructions on how to make and store formula for later use. If air swallowing occurs during the feeding, you can often hear it in the form of loud, gulping sounds during the feeding. If this happens, be sure to double-check that the nipple size isn't too fast for your baby.

Seek Help

Some babies who struggle to eat stop enjoying the process and can develop an oral aversion. Feeding has become a lot of work for both the parents and the baby at this point. Any discomfort from dysphagia can contribute to a negative experience during feeding. After all, gagging and choking do not feel good!

If a baby starts to cry at the sight of a bottle or gags when offered the nipple, she may start to take less volume or refuse to eat altogether. This results in an enormous amount of pressure, stress, and concern for parents. Parents know their baby needs to receive nutrition so may sometimes resort to force-feeding, possibly in gentler forms and difficult to recognize. Some examples include

- Offering your baby the bottle more than a few times in a feeding despite refusals
- Prolonging the feeding for up to an hour or more, after your baby has already indicated she is done eating
- Rocking your baby into a sleepy state so she eats with less of a struggle

It is hard work to help a baby with an oral aversion to learn to enjoy eating again, but it can be done! However, it may be more easily achieved with professional guidance from a feeding specialist. If these strategies do not help your baby feed better, you notice coughing or choking, or your baby seems to be actively avoiding feeding, raise these concerns with your primary care physician to seek further guidance. Feeding plans need to be individualized, based on development and research, and a specialist can help review all the components of what your baby needs to be successful.

Feeding Milestones

A baby receives his primary nourishment and hydration from breastfeeding or bottle-feeding for at least the first 12 months after birth. Readiness for the introduction of pureed solids and cup drinking is based on posture, digestion, and swallowing development for these transitions.

The current standard is to begin offering pureed solid foods at around 6 months of age. Your baby should be showing some readiness to sit upright. Look at your baby's head control to see if she is ready. She should be able to move her head freely from her trunk so she can look around without effort. Trunk control allows her to sit upright without leaning forward to prop on her arms (Figure 10.6). In the high chair, she should not be leaning on the tray for support or leaning to the side to help her sit upright (Figure 10.7). When a baby is sitting better, she won't have to concentrate on sitting well in the high chair. Instead, she can focus on using her mouth to eat! For babies with a history of fussy or colicky behaviors, introducing solid foods can make parents a little nervous. The following tips can set you and your baby up for success:

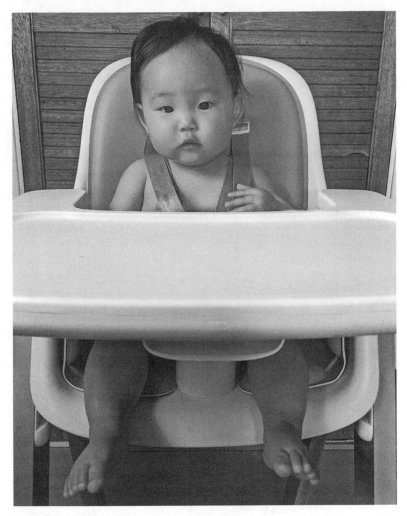

Figure 10.6. Baby sitting in a supportive high chair.

- Use a supportive high chair with a high back and straps and harness. You can use rolled towels to help if need be (Figure 10.8).
- Start with very smooth, pureed foods, such as stage 1 jars or infant cereals. Be careful not to make foods too thick or lumpy if they are homemade.
- Allow your baby to just touch and play with the food before trying to feed him. Set it on the tray and watch him enjoy exploring the new textures!
- If your baby loves to mouth, offer some small dipper infant spoons and teethers while he plays with the food. He can get some indirect tastes and see what interesting new stuff in his mouth feels and tastes like.

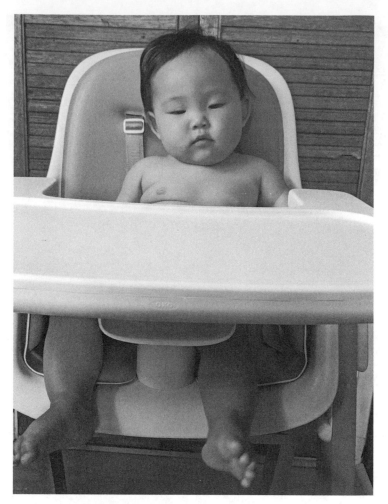

Figure 10.7. Baby leaning in the high chair.

- ❧ End the meal before he gets upset. Watch for him to start to drop or lean; he may be tired from sitting in the chair or may start to look around the room out of boredom.
- ❧ Remember, he isn't eating for hunger with pureed solids at this point, only for learning. It doesn't matter how much he takes.
- ❧ Let your baby get messy! He's having fun and learning that new food can be enjoyable.
- ❧ Never, ever "sneak" bites in if he opens his mouth to yawn or smile. It could startle or even cause him to choke.

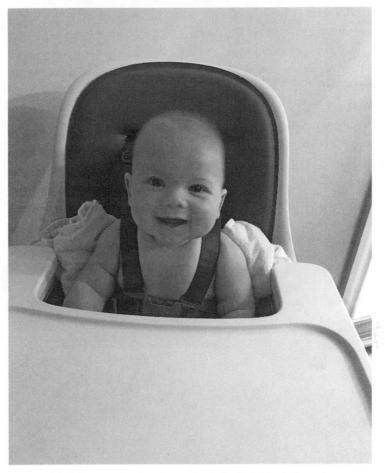

Figure 10.8. Baby supported with towel rolls in the high chair.

Did You Know?

Dipper spoons are shorter than regular infant spoons and are often made of silicone or a soft texture. They are for babies to use to taste foods independently. The wider handle is easier for them to hold and because they are short, babies are less likely to gag themselves.

The strategies in this chapter are simply guidelines. If you feel your baby may have dysphagia or that you need more guidance with feeding, discuss it with your primary care physician. Ask about a possible evaluation with a speech-language pathologist who specializes in infant feeding.

Remember, just as your baby is learning to eat, you are learning to help him. This may feel like a marathon on some days, but hang in there! It helps to know you aren't alone. Feeding challenges are not uncommon, and there are trained feeding specialists available for extra guidance. All your hard work and dedication to overcoming these challenges will be worth it. For one mom, resolving her son's feeding issues helped with bonding so much that she said, "I finally enjoy my baby!"

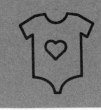

Chapter 11

Infantile Colic: Can Diet Help?

Every parent thinks about their baby's nutrition! What we feed our babies provides the crucial building block to their health. You've heard the phrase "breast is best"; it's true: breast milk provides the energy, protein, vitamins, and minerals your baby needs to grow and thrive. But why is your baby so fussy if breast milk is the best? Are you worried you are eating something that affects your milk or that your milk is lacking something? Or are you shopping around for the perfect "no fuss" infant formula? There are so many on the market; how do you choose the best nutrition for your baby? If a diet therapy works for one baby, how do you know it will work for *your* baby? Let's take a careful look at how diet can affect infantile colic.

Safety First

Before making any changes to your or your baby's diet, always consult your primary care physician first. Together you can determine what diet plan is best for you and your baby and your doctor can monitor both of your plans.

Low Allergen/Elimination Diets

While Breastfeeding

Some breastfeeding moms request to try or are recommended a low-allergen or elimination diet to see if it will soothe their colicky baby. Unless there is blood or mucous present in your baby's stool, or a strong family history of food allergies, it is best not to blame fussiness on maternal intake. If you are breastfeeding and feel strongly about trying an elimination diet, just know that it can be challenging, and it is a good idea to discuss your diet with a dietitian, to make sure you are consuming the nutrients you and your baby need. True allergic colitis is typically due to dairy and/or soy, so it is a good idea to start with only eliminating these foods instead of all major food allergens. If you decide to eliminate cow's milk from your diet, adding an alternate form of milk to your diet, that is fortified with calcium and vitamin D is strongly recommended. There are many types of alternative milks on the market; soy, almond, hemp, oat, and coconut milk are the most popular varieties. Many of the alternative milks contain very little protein, so it is important you get enough protein from other foods such as meats, beans, eggs, nuts, and seeds. You should also take a calcium supplement that contains vitamin D, in addition to your prenatal vitamins.

Eliminating all major food allergens from your diet, including dairy, soy, wheat, eggs, peanuts, tree nuts, and fish, is not a typical recommendation as a colic treatment. A diet this limited would not only be very hard to maintain but would likely not be healthy or complete—and might reduce your supply of breast milk. If you have strong feelings that these foods are causing your baby distress, discuss this with your dietitian or doctor before removing them from your diet.

If you do not see any changes in your baby's fussiness after 2 weeks of allergen elimination, it is recommended to add the eliminated food(s) back to your diet. Add the eliminated foods back to your diet one at a time each week and take note if any of symptoms return. This way you can determine which food allergen causes your baby the most discomfort and continue to avoid it for the duration of your breastfeeding experience.

For Formula-Fed Babies

There is some evidence that hypoallergenic formulas may help some bottle-fed babies with colic. These formulas have been *hydrolyzed,* meaning the protein has broken down into tiny components. Babies who are sensitive to these proteins may have less of a reaction to these pieces than to the larger protein molecules. These studies indicate that babies on these formulas cry and fuss less than babies taking a standard cow's milk–based formula.

As with elimination diets for breastfeeding, try the hydrolyzed formula for 2 weeks. If your baby does not seem better, revert to a standard formula.

Food Avoidance During Breastfeeding

Breastfeeding moms may often wonder if their baby is fussy due to the foods they eat. Breast milk is the perfect nutrition for a baby, no matter what the mother eats. A breastfeeding mother's body knows exactly what nutrition her baby needs at every stage of development.

Most babies can tolerate spicy or gassy foods such as beans, broccoli, cabbage, or brussels sprouts passed through breast milk. But if you notice that your baby seems to have excess gas or diarrhea every time you eat a specific food, avoid it for a few weeks to see if symptoms improve. Cook the vegetables before you eat them too; raw veggies sometimes can be more troublesome than cooked.

It may be helpful to keep a log of your diet and your baby's symptoms. It's easy to eliminate 1 or 2 foods if you think they might be causing a problem and see if it helps.

Probiotics

Probiotics are live bacteria in the digestive system that help to keep the gut healthy. There are many different kinds of probiotics, each one having its own effect on the body. There is quite a lot of research on the effects of probiotics for gastrointestinal disorders, such as diarrhea or irritable bowel syndrome.

Most recent studies do not show that probiotics have a positive effect on infantile colic. However, there is one specific strain of probiotic that has been shown to help with gassiness and fussiness in breastfed babies. The probiotic strain, *Lactobacillus reuteri*, is found naturally in the digestive system, urinary tract, skin, and breast milk. One study showed babies given *L reuteri* for 1 week cried less than babies given simethicone (gas drops).

It is not clear why this seems to help breastfed babies but not bottle-fed babies, and the question is still being studied. One theory is that breastfed babies have different microorganisms (*gut microbiota*) in their digestive systems, so they react differently to the probiotic. It is also important to take note that many premade infant formulas contain prebiotics, which can alter the gut microbiota and may lessen the effects of the probiotic.

There are few reported side effects when giving probiotics to babies, the most common being excess gas. If you want to try giving your baby a probiotic, check with your pediatrician first. Probiotics might not be safe to give to some babies, especially babies with lower immune systems. Read the label to make sure the product you give has the *L reuteri* strain listed and follow the dosing instructions carefully.

Prebiotics

Prebiotics, or *oligosaccharides,* have been introduced into most infant formulas over the past decade in the United States. These are carbohydrates found naturally in breast milk. Prebiotics are a type of dietary fiber that feed into the good bacteria of the gut to help keep a healthy digestive system. They serve as "food" for the probiotics. The most common prebiotic added to foods comes from chicory root, a plant in the dandelion family. Chicory root contains the prebiotic inulin, which you may see on the label of many lower-sugar, higher-fiber foods. Other foods that naturally contain prebiotics include onions, leeks, bananas, asparagus, garlic, and legumes.

While probiotics tend to show positive effects only in breastfed babies, prebiotics in infant formulas have produced some positive outcomes, such as improved frequency and consistency of bowel movements. This is attributed to the increased amount of "good bacteria" in these babies' guts, compared with the guts of babies on standard formula without added prebiotics. Prebiotic-containing infant formulas have been proven to be safe; therefore, it would be a simple diet therapy to try without any side effects.

Herbal Therapies

Although we do not necessarily recommend or endorse herbal therapies, it is important to discuss and educate parents on what they are and some of the common concerns with using them for colic relief. These anecdotal "remedies" are popular on the internet and among desperate parents trying to find the answer to soothe their colicky baby. Please use the following as a guide to help you understand the concerns of using popular alternative dietary therapies for your baby. If you are interested in trying a therapy, consult your pediatrician before beginning.

Fennel Tea

Fennel tea or oil is often suggested for gas relief and colic because of its reputation as a "natural laxative." The fennel plant belongs to the parsley family. A few studies suggest that fennel tea stimulates bowel movements by increasing the movement in the gut, which may help with colic.

If you are considering fennel tea as a therapy for colic, it should only be given to infants older than 6 months. Note that it is not recommended to give anything other than breast milk or infant formula to babies younger than 6 months. If a baby drinks too much tea, she may not take in enough milk to be properly nourished. Too much water (or tea) can also be dangerous, as it can dilute the bloodstream and interfere with normal body functions. If you are interested in trying fennel tea, remember to get your use of it approved by your primary care physician first. Give only small amounts of the tea (<4 oz/d) and, of course, make sure it has cooled before you give it to your baby.

Gripe Water

Gripe water is another herbal remedy marketed for infantile colic. It is typically made of a blend of different herbs, such as fennel, ginger, chamomile, licorice, cinnamon, and lemon balm. This, or any other herbal remedy, is not regulated by the US Food and Drug Administration, and there are no standards for quality or dosing, so check with your primary care physician before using. Any prepared herbal product, such as gripe water, may also contain extra ingredients, such as sugar, alcohol, or baking soda, which could have unwanted or unhealthy effects. Therefore, gripe water is not recommended for infants at this time

Lactase Treatment/Lactose Intolerance

There are infant drops on the market for lactose intolerance. There is little to no evidence that they actually work for babies with colic. These drops contain *lactase,* an enzyme normally produced in the small intestine. Lactase breaks down *lactose,* the sugar in milk. People who do not have enough lactase in their system to digest lactose develop lactose intolerance. When they eat dairy products, they may have bloating, cramps, and diarrhea.

All babies are born with lactase in their intestines, so it is very rare for a baby to be intolerant to lactose. Lactase enzymes gradually decrease as children grow. Lactose intolerance typically only develops after age 3 years, or perhaps not until the teen and adult years.

At this time there is no current evidence that shows lactase treatment will help your baby with colic. There are some cases of actual lactase deficiency in babies, but this is rare and typically caused by health problems such as an intestinal problem, chemotherapy, or a birth defect. In these situations, your pediatrician or specialist would be the best source for help before trying any commercial products.

Colic Relief Therapies

While some babies might benefit from alternative therapies, the research does not offer any conclusive answers. Supplements such as fennel tea and gripe water have been studied, but there are concerns about the safety and effectiveness of these unregulated products. The recent research on probiotics and prebiotics shows promise but is not complete and shouldn't be considered a single solution for colic.

The elimination of certain foods and/or allergens from a breastfeeding mother's diet can be a safe way to rule out intolerances but is not recommended unless there are definite signs of allergy, as a diet elimination could cause unnecessary stress on the mother. If you do decide to eliminate foods from your diet while breastfeeding, it is very important that you maintain a healthy, well-rounded diet from all food groups to be sure you receive all the nutrients you and your baby need. It is also important to make only one change at time, so you can determine what is helping.

If you consider trying any of these approaches, talk to your primary care physician first to make sure you are making safe choices for both you and your baby.

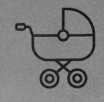

Chapter 12

Understanding Your Baby's Postural Control

Typical development in a growing baby is an amazing process to watch. You give birth to this little baby, who starts out learning how to cope with the overwhelming sensory world outside the womb (including the effects of gravity!), and then in a year or so, she is walking all over the place. How did she do that?

Many things affect the process of typical development. Pediatric literature talks about the interplay between heredity and the environment, or nature versus nurture. One is not more important than the other; they work together to influence development in terms of personality, intelligence, and overall brain development.

- *Heredity.* This is based on the genes your baby inherits from both parents that express certain traits such as hair color, height, body type, etc. You cannot control heredity.
- *Environment.* This is what babies see, hear, and feel (both movement and touch) as you handle them during daily care. Early home environments have long-term effects on the development of your baby. You have the ability to control your environment to best meet the needs of your baby.

Important Developmental Tasks and Positions

Typical development can vary quite a bit from baby to baby. Some babies sit at 4 months and some not until 7 months; some babies walk at 9 months and some not until 14 months. This is all within the range of typical development.

When babies are born, they tend to be in a flexed position due to being in this position in the uterus. This is called *physiological flexion* or the *fetal position*. We learned earlier that flexion and midline is a very organizing position. We need to think of this when handling all babies, and especially fussy babies. This flexion decreases as they start acclimating to gravity and start developing new motor skills. All babies tend to follow the same sequence but at different rates. Babies gain control of their head first, and then their trunk. They need strong core strength before they start to use their arms and legs in a coordinated way. Typical development also involves *postural control*. We all move in 3 different planes of movement: laterally (side to side), forward and backward, and with rotation (turning). The development of rotation is what allows babies to roll, come to a sitting position, and walk. Having your baby lie on her tummy regularly (*tummy time*) is critical for developing her postural control. Table 12.1 lists the critical developmental tasks during your baby's first 6 months.

From looking at all the developmental tasks in Table 12.1, you can see how important it is for babies to be free on the floor on their tummy, back, and side and not in baby-holding equipment (see Chapter 8 and the "A Word About Baby-Holding Equipment" box later in this chapter). If they are in baby-holding equipment too long, postural control cannot develop in a typical way. Babies use their trunk, neck, arms, and legs much less while they are in baby-holding devices. Being confined in this equipment also limits their sensory experience and exploration of their bodies.

Back Position

Lying on the back is good to do at times and helps babies develop important movement patterns like hands together at midline, hands to mouth, hands to knees, and hands to feet. Babies also start to reach for toys dangling from an activity gym. When your baby spends time on her back, make sure that her head does not show a preference in turning only to 1 side or tilting with 1 ear closer to the shoulder than the other ear. Her head should turn from 1 side to the other. By the time they are 3 months old, most babies should be able to hold their head in the middle by themselves. They won't gain much head control when being on their back, but they do gain freedom of movement of the head and neck. If babies spend too much time on their backs, they could possibly get a flat spot on the back of their head. (See the Tummy Time section later in this chapter for more information).

Table 12.1. Critical Developmental Tasks (First 6 Months)

Newborn	Full-term babies are born with physiological flexion, which is observed in all positions
	Nonpurposeful, jerky, or random movements of the arms and legs
	Strong grasp reflex on your finger or a toy
	While on his back, his head is often to 1 side or the other, not always held in the middle
	While on his tummy, he leans on 1 cheek or the other; does not lift his head a lot
	Hands are often fisted
1–2 mo	The nonpurposeful, jerky, random movements now have a wider excursion of movement with both the arms and legs
	Head lags when pulled to sitting position from her back
	Lifts her head off your shoulder
	Head bobs in supported sitting position
	Begins to hold head straight in all positions
	On her tummy, can lift her head to turn to the other side
	Puts hands to mouth
3–5 mo	Puts hands to knees and to feet while on his back
	Rolls to the side from his back
	Starts to roll from tummy to back
	Lifts head and holds it erect when on his tummy
	Spends time on his tummy on bent elbows
	Holds his head straight in all positions
	Occasionally props on his arms when in a sitting position
	Begins to reach for toys while on his back
6 mo	Rolls from back to tummy
	Pushes up on straight elbows when on her tummy
	May move to a hands and knees position
	Sits independently with either arms propped on the surface or sits tall without arm support

Side-lying Position

Lying on the side is a typical developmental position, and the benefits of this position are often overlooked by parents who are not aware how important this play position is. Babies can roll to their side purposefully but not until 4 or 5 months of age. Sometimes a baby will curl up in a ball and accidentally roll to the side earlier than that, which may be an effort to self-soothe. If he rolls to his side, you can leave him there as long as he is awake and supervised. This is a great position for babies, as it helps to reduce the startle reflex, moves their hands to midline, keeps their head centered in the middle, and avoids pressure on the back of the head, which can cause flattening. If your baby seems to prefer mostly looking to 1 side, side-lying helps balance the body. Make sure your baby lies on both sides during side-lying play. Babies start growing out of the side-lying position when they start rolling a lot and don't want to stay here long. Take advantage of this position with younger babies.

Did You Know?

Physical and occupational therapists have been using the side-lying position therapeutically for years to help achieve developmental milestones in children who are developmentally delayed. In recent years, this position has been taught to parents of typically developing babies to give other play options besides placing babies in equipment or on their tummies. Due to the Back to Sleep campaign parents were reluctant to put their babies on their tummies at all, so they ended up using baby equipment. The side-lying position offers parents an alternate play position to keep them out of containers.

Tummy Time

The importance of tummy time cannot be overstated. Being on the tummy is a very organizing position for babies. It helps the development of head and neck control as well as arm strength. It is also the first step toward mastering more challenging tasks such as army crawling (tummy down) and creeping on hands and knees. It is critical for development of typical motor patterns; babies need to be on their tummies to practice those developmental milestones as much as possible. Awake and supervised tummy time is safe and beneficial in many ways and can actually start the day the baby gets home from the hospital!

A Word About Baby-Holding Equipment

Baby-holding equipment includes swings, gliders, bouncers, rockers, infant seats, floor seats, vibrating chairs, jumpers, strollers, floor sitters, saucers, infant recliners, infant nappers, rocking sleepers, and more, and there are new products coming out all the time. This can be truly overwhelming! With all this equipment on the market, how do you know what to buy? What will help your baby, what is a convenience, is your baby safe in any of them, and what might be harmful?

Truthfully, most households only need 1 or 2 pieces of baby-holding equipment, if that. They are fine to put your baby in briefly, such as while you cook dinner, but should not be used for hours on end. The overuse of them can be harmful, causing poor head shape, developmental delays, and restriction for babies in exploring their sensory world. There are virtually no developmental advantages to these pieces of equipment. Using jumpers won't help your baby stand or walk early and, in fact, may inhibit the desire to walk. Some babies are put in jumpers and saucers too early, when they don't have the postural (head or trunk) control to maintain being upright, so they just lean to the side, which is not a comfortable position to be in. Inclined baby-holding equipment is never recommended for sleeping, even if labeled as a napper or sleeper.

Buy only 1 or 2 that you like and that fit well in your house, but keep in mind that babies can thrive without using any of these pieces of equipment. Babies also grow out of them very quickly. The American Academy of Pediatrics does not recommend the use of walkers and recommends no more than 2 hours a day in baby-holding equipment and no more than 15 minutes at a time. Play mats and tummy time mats are OK as long as they don't restrict your baby's movement. Make sure that a tummy time pillow is not too high and is comfortable for your baby. Play yards are great to keep babies safe from pets or siblings.

We recommend that by 3 months of age your baby spend 60 minutes per day on his tummy, and up to 90 minutes for those older than 3 months (obviously not all at once, but several short sessions throughout the day). Research shows that babies who have less tummy time (and more time in holding equipment) score lower on developmental tests. Every time your baby is awake, he should spend

Car Safety Seat Guidelines

Appropriate use of approved car seats is critical for all travel in the car. The American Academy of Pediatrics "...recommends that all infants ride rear facing starting with their first ride home from the hospital. All infants and toddlers should ride in a rear-facing seat until they reach the highest weight or height allowed by their car safety seat manufacturer. Most convertible seats have limits that will allow children to ride rear facing for 2 years or more. When infants outgrow their rear-facing–only seat, a convertible seat installed rear facing is needed. All parents can benefit from getting installation help from a CPST [child passenger safety technician] to ensure that their child's seat is properly installed."

Source: American Academy of Pediatrics. Rear-facing car seats for infants and toddlers. HealthyChildren.org. Updated February 24, 2020. Accessed November 5, 2020. https://www.healthy children.org/English/safety-prevention/on-the-go/Pages/Rear-Facing-Car-Seats-for-Infants-Toddlers.aspx

some time on his tummy. Start with only a couple minutes at a time as tolerated, while ensuring supervision at all times. Remember, back to sleep, tummy to play. Prior to the 1990s most babies slept on their tummies. Although recommendations to sleep on their back drastically decreased the number of sudden infant death syndrome (SIDS) deaths, the rates of plagiocephaly (or flattening of the back of the head) have also increased. Plagiocephaly is not a life-threatening problem, and the asymmetrical head shape is generally only a cosmetic problem. It generally gets better on its own as your baby spends more time upright. However, it can be largely prevented by starting awake tummy time early on and then gradually increasing the amount of time spent in awake tummy time with the activities outlined in this chapter. You can also decrease the amount of time in baby-holding equipment as we discussed previously in this chapter. If you are concerned about your baby's head position or head shape, talk to your primary care physician and consider undergoing a physical therapy evaluation. Some babies may benefit from wearing a helmet (*cranial orthosis*) to help with their head shape; your physical therapist can help you get to the correct resources if needed. It is important to start early when you see a problem with your baby's head shape or head preference. Early physical therapy helps reduce a baby's head preference to a certain side, helps your baby develop more symmetrically, stimulates motor development, and even helps to avoid the need for helmet therapy. Sometimes, helmet therapy is indicated, depending on your baby's age.

Early helmet therapy results in a shorter duration of wearing the helmet as well as having a better chance of improving head shape.

When it comes to baby equipment, be choosy about what you really need and forget all the other bells and whistles; remember, being on the floor to explore is best!

Positioning to Help With Postural Control

When placing newborns on their tummy they can be a little top-heavy, meaning their bottom is higher than their head, their head is usually leaning to 1 side, and they lean on their cheek. This is the ideal position! They do not lift their heads much at this age except maybe to turn it to the other side. It is important for your baby to be in this position without a lot of support because she needs to learn how to use her muscles to lift her head, free an arm, and shift side to side. If you always put your baby on a nursing pillow or those tummy time mats, she doesn't have the opportunity to learn this. With young babies, you can also do tummy time on your chest. Lie down in a recliner or flat on the floor. Place your baby on your chest with her head facing you. We call this the Front to Front position (Figure 12.1). Here she will begin to learn how to lift her head, but sometimes she will just put her head down, usually on 1 cheek—which is fine and still considered tummy time! Another tummy time position for younger babies is the arm drape or the Hanging Out position. This is when

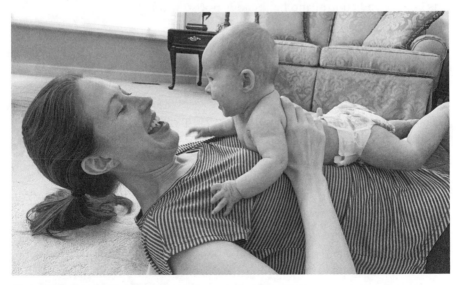

Figure 12.1. Front to Front.

you hold the baby on your forearm facing the floor (Figures 12.2 and 12.3). Your baby's head can be near your elbow, or it can be supported in your hand. Either version is a great position for fussy babies (see the "CALM Positions for Fussy Babies" section later in this chapter). This position is a favorite among dads, as their forearms are typically longer than mom's! If you haven't tried tummy time yet, don't worry—it's not too late! Every time your baby is awake, supervise tummy time on the floor or in the alternate tummy time positions listed later in this section. This may be difficult for some babies at first. If your baby starts fussing, try to distract her. Offer something interesting to look at, such as a mirror, an exciting toy, a sibling, or the other parent. This will keep her there longer and entertained. Don't just place her on her tummy with nothing to look at—this should be fun playtime. Anytime you engage in tummy time and she starts to fuss, try rolling her out of this position, playing a little, and then rolling her back…she'll get it eventually! Sometimes it helps to start her on her back and help her roll slowly side to side and then, eventually, roll her all the way to her tummy. This is a less abrupt transition than just placing her straight down on her tummy. Bottom line: we don't want her to just lie on her tummy and fuss and cry. Colicky babies do enough fussing and crying! As your baby grows older and has more head control, you can do many other alternative tummy time positions with all the same benefits. Being on the tummy is a much more organizing position than being on her back, where she startles more.

Here are several alternate tummy time positions to use when your baby has better head control and her head is not so wobbly:

- *Front to Front.* Place your older baby on your chest while you are in a recliner or on the floor; he is just a little heavier! Your baby will lift his head and look around, gaining good control, and it is fun being so close to you! (See Figure 12.1.)
- *A Little Boost.* Lay your baby on his tummy with a blanket rolled up underneath his armpits (Figure 12.4). (A nursing pillow may be a little too high.) This gives him a little boost so he doesn't have to work so hard. It helps to keep his elbows under his shoulders, which makes it easier to lift his head. Make sure to remove the roll when your baby can maintain his elbows under his shoulders by himself.
- *Look Me in the Eye.* This is a fun position! Lie down on the floor on your tummy and face your baby while he is on his tummy. Support his elbows with your hands so he feels secure and then lift up his head (Figure 12.5). If his arms are too far back, he will struggle to lift his head.

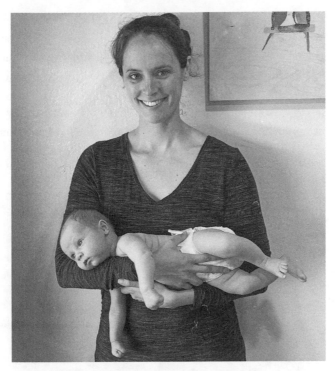

Figure 12.2. Hanging Out. (Using both of your arms to hold your baby, this pose is when your baby's head is cradled in the crease of your elbow.)

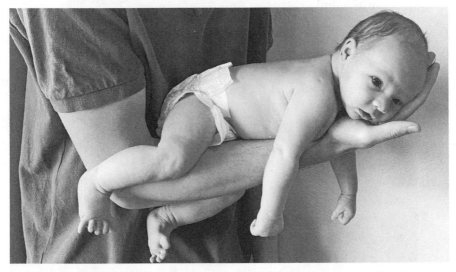

Figure 12.3. Hanging Out. (Using one of your arms, this pose is when your baby's head is supported by your hand. It is a favorite pose for many dads, who typically have longer forearms.)

❧ *Crisscross Tummy Time.* While you sit on the floor in a pretzel position, place your baby on your bent knee (Figure 12.6). Have toys or something else to look at available. Support him with your hand on his back or at his upper arms so he feels secure. Do this on both of your legs to change the position.

❧ *Hold Me Tight.* Hold your baby while you stand or kneel, tummy down, with you supporting his arms and his bottom "sitting" on your belly (Figure 12.7). Walk around the house singing, dancing, and showing him the world!

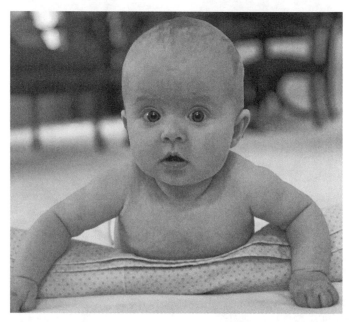

Figure 12.4. A Little Boost.

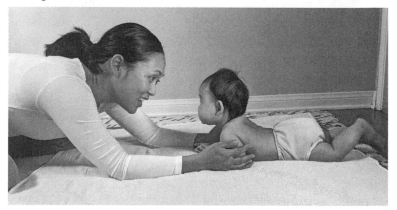

Figure 12.5. Look Me in the Eye.

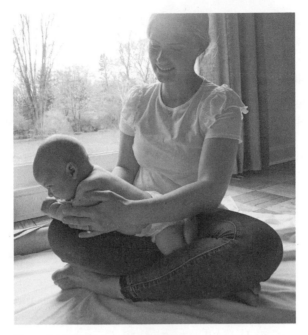

Figure 12.6. Crisscross Tummy Time.

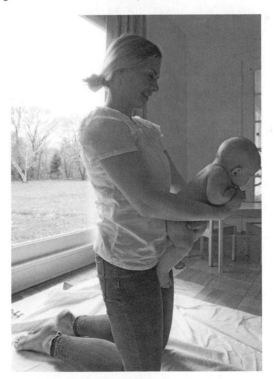

Figure 12.7. Hold Me Tight.

Baby Yoga Poses

Consider engaging in some baby yoga poses that can help with endurance for tummy time. Baby yoga poses are just fun touch and movement activities to do with your baby. These are playful and engaging, and most babies love them! See what your baby likes, but don't force anything. If your baby doesn't like it the first time, try again at another time. The best time to do baby yoga is when your baby is in the quiet alert state of arousal. Don't engage in baby yoga when your baby is fussy, as this may overstimulate him. You also don't want to do a lot of movement activities too close to bedtime because this may arouse him too much, and we want to help calm your baby before bedtime. Some days you may have time for a couple of these activities in a row; other days that might be too much. Remember to watch your baby's cues to see what he likes and doesn't like. These positions and activities include

- *Hug a Knee.* This position is for a younger, smaller baby. Place your baby draped on your bent knee, his head at your knee and bottom toward your stomach. You can raise and lower your knee to change the support as needed as well as to provide a gentle movement. You can also massage his back in this position (Figure 12.8).

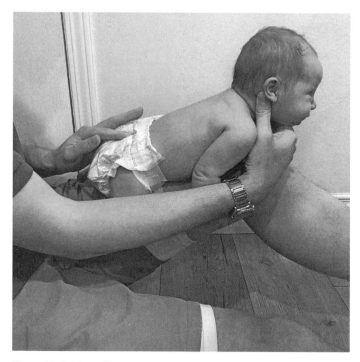

Figure 12.8. Hug a Knee.

- *Roll With Me Baby.* Lie on your back with your baby on your chest, put both arms around your baby, and then roll slowly from side to side while holding onto your baby. Just roll a small amount, not all the way to your side (Figure 12.9).
- *Tummy Time Incline.* Sit on the floor with your legs straight and cross your ankles so there is a little incline when you place your baby on his tummy across your thighs. He can be on his elbows or with his arms dangling. Make sure your baby has some degree of head control before trying this position (Figures 12.10 and 12.11).

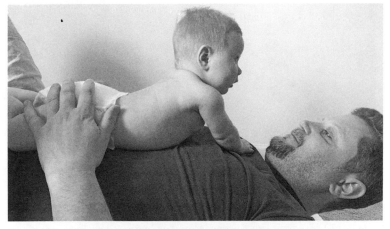

Figure 12.9. Roll With Me Baby.

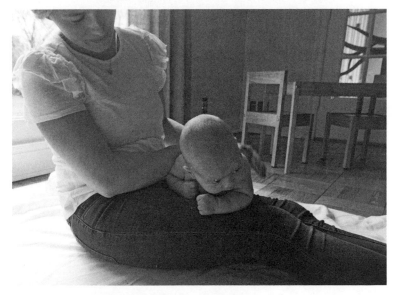

Figure 12.10. Tummy Time Incline (on elbows).

- *Airplane Baby.* This is for an older, stronger baby with good head and trunk control. Lie on your back and bend your legs. Place your baby on your shins and raise and lower him slowly (Figure 12.12). (Watch out for spit up or drool!)
- *Swinging Baby.* This is another position for a stronger baby. Hold him with your hands around his rib cage facing down, looking at the floor, while you bend forward. You can swing back and forth a little if he likes it (Figure 12.13).

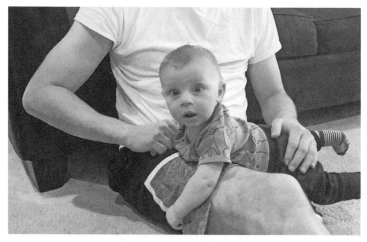

Figure 12.11. Tummy Time Incline (arms dangling).

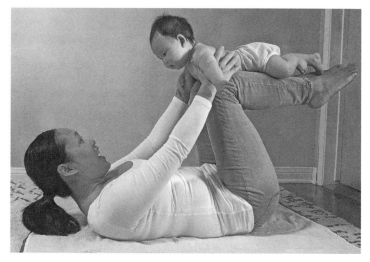

Figure 12.12. Airplane Baby.

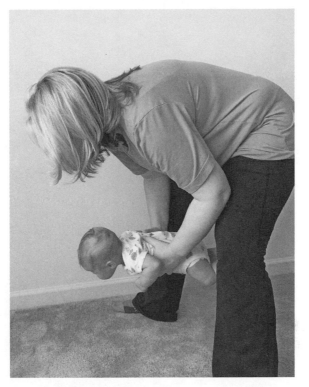

Figure 12.13. Swinging Baby.

- *Baby on a Boat Pose.* Again, this is a pose for a stronger baby. It is a universal yoga pose for adults, but you can enjoy this with your baby too. Sit on your bottom with your knees bent and feet on the floor. Hold your baby firmly on your shins (Figure 12.14). You can stay there or lean back and lift your legs so they are horizontal to the floor. You can also put him on your thighs facing out and hold him firmly in that position (Figure 12.15).

> "*My daughter loves all the baby yoga positions. It is a fun, bonding activity that also teaches her how to be mobile and gives her new ways to see the world. She smiles the entire time!*"
>
> Mother of a 3-month-old

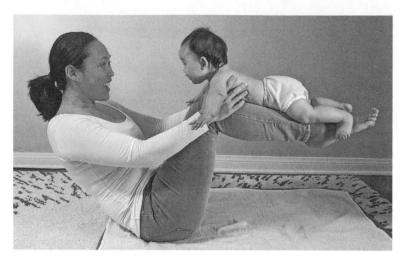

Figure 12.14. Baby on a Boat (baby facing in).

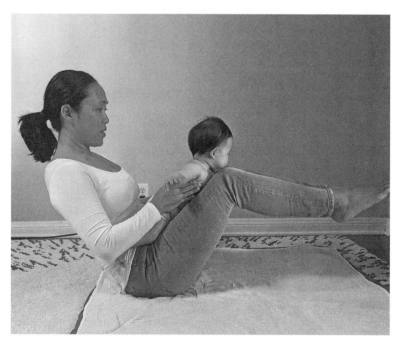

Figure 12.15. Baby on a Boat (baby facing out).

Anyone can do tummy time with your baby: grandparents, sitters, child care providers, or older siblings. Show them how to do it safely and which ways your baby likes tummy time the best. Once your baby practices more often, she will love being on her tummy, and before you know it, she'll be crawling!

Baby Wearing and Colic Carries

While freedom of movement is critical for healthy motor development, sometimes feeling contained serves a purpose when done deliberately and thoughtfully. Fussy or high-need babies like to be held, worn, and carried. Fussy babies often extend and arch more than typical babies. Being held gives them boundaries and helps them be contained and more organized. (Remember, flexion is organizing!) "Baby wearing" is a wonderful option to carry your baby. Helpful tools such as slings and front-wearing carriers (there is even a double carrier for twins!) allow you to have your hands free so you can get something done while wearing your baby.

There are several benefits to both you and your baby when you wear him. Your hands are free to tend to something else. It reminds your baby of being in the womb; it contains your baby; and it offers an attachment or closeness with you. All of these are great for interaction, and the motion while you walk around may have a calming effect. When you carry your baby close, practice deep breathing. This not only calms you but leads your baby into a nice, slow breathing pattern that calms him too. When you wear or carry your baby, be very careful of his head position to avoid head and neck hypertension. And remember, you should always be able to see your baby's face. Never cook or handle hot liquids or sharp objects when you wear your baby; make sure your posture is good and not causing any strain on you. Finally, don't bend over; this is bad for your back and could make your baby fall out. Always squat if you have to pick something up. Try to switch your baby's head position from side to side or wear him on different sides so he develops equally on both sides.

Hip Dysplasia

Baby wearing is becoming increasingly popular; however, there are some risks with regard to hip development. *Hip dysplasia* is a hip condition that can occur in utero. Proper hip positioning in baby carriers, in baby wearing devices, and while being swaddled is very important to good hip development and helps prevent hip dysplasia. The International Hip Dysplasia Institute states that short-term use of baby carriers and baby wearing is unlikely to have any effect on hip development. As with most things, moderation is key!

CALM Positions for Fussy Babies

For younger babies who have not developed good head control yet, and also for smaller babies who are not too heavy, try the following hold or carries:

- *Hanging Out.* This is the same as the tummy time position pictured in Figures 12.2 and 12.3 earlier in this chapter. For a gassy or colicky baby, make sure your hand is on his belly to give warmth and support. This is easier when your baby's head is near your elbow. With a fussy baby you can add a gentle bounce to your walk to provide some good movement sensation.
- *Baby Bundle.* Hold your baby in a sitting position facing outward with legs bent, hands together and close to mouth, and leaning a little forward (Figures 12.16 and 12.17). This keeps him in that flexed position and hands to midline, which, as we learned, is very organizing. Walk around while holding him. As you have probably discovered, sometimes fussy babies won't let you sit down!

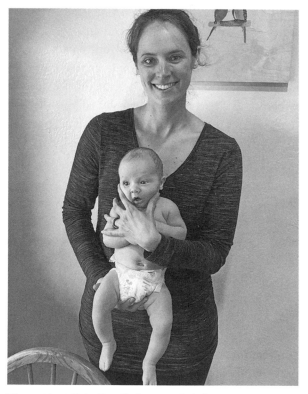

Figure 12.16. Baby Bundle (younger baby).

 📌 *Happy Baby, Happy Mama.* This is the Happy Baby Pose (see the Other Developmentally Beneficial Positions section later in this chapter) but on your lap with hands together (Figure 12.18). It is also a nice flexed position. It is a fun position to sing little songs and enjoy your baby!

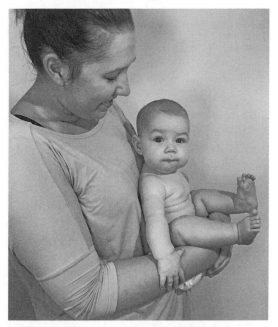

Figure 12.17. Baby Bundle (older baby).

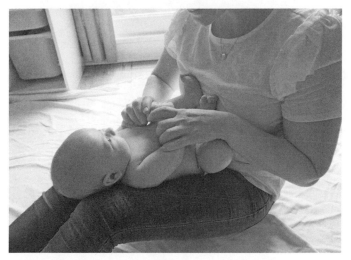

Figure 12.18. Happy Baby, Happy Mama.

᪐ *Hello World Hold.* This is for a slightly older, heavier baby who has good head control. Put your arm around his chest with his arms over the top of yours. Then, with your other hand, come from behind (or from the front) and hold his diaper that way (Figure 12.19). Walk around and let him see the world.

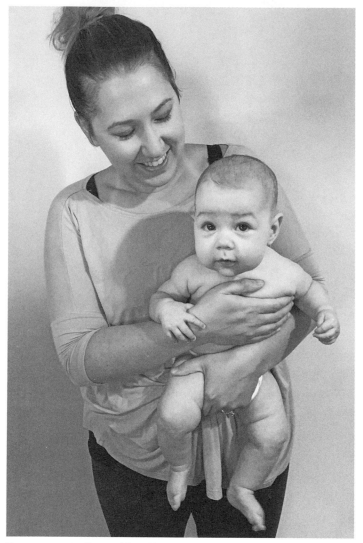

Figure 12.19. Hello World Hold.

✍ *Cradle Hold.* This is just as it sounds. Hold your baby cradled in your arms so he is slightly reclined. However, make sure to keep his hands together, and don't let the arm closest to you go behind your back. Remember, flexion and hands together are organizing (Figure 12.20).

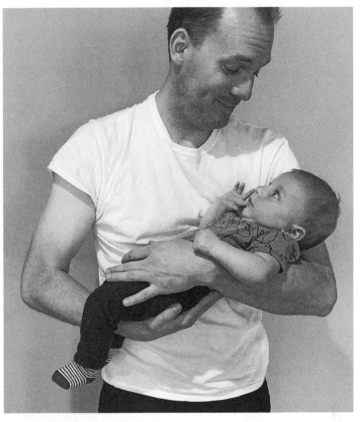

Figure 12.20. Cradle Hold.

> "Having so many different ways to hold my crying baby made me feel so much better, like I was actually doing something. I could sometimes even stop the crying! And for the first time she [my daughter] started letting me hold her."
>
> Father of a 2-month-old fussy baby

Other Developmentally Beneficial Positions

There are other developmentally beneficial positions besides tummy time that may help calm and organize your baby; most of them include flexion and midline.

    Side-lying (both sides, with or without a blanket roll). You can help your baby become more stable by bending his knee and crossing his top leg over his bottom and planting his foot on the floor (Figure 12.21). You may have to help hold him at his hip.

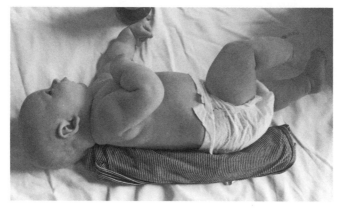

Figure 12.21. Side-lying (with a blanket roll).

    Happy Baby Pose. This is a universal pose in yoga. Have your baby lie down on her back and help her grab her feet, right foot to right hand, left foot to left hand, and slowly roll her side to side. You can also hold this position static (Figure 12.22).

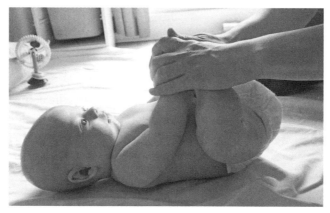

Figure 12.22. Happy Baby Pose.

➤ *Nested Baby.* While your baby is on her back roll up baby blankets and put them on either side of her body (Figure 12.23); this helps to reduce the startle because it supports her arms. You can leave the rolls like that on the diaper-changing table too, so she doesn't startle as much when changing her diaper.

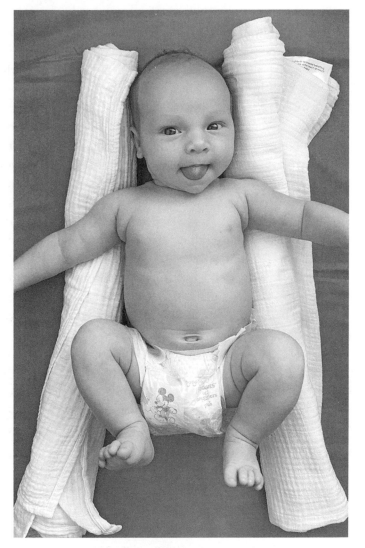

Figure 12.23. Nested Baby.

Swaddling

There are many benefits to swaddling, so don't stop once you come home from the hospital. The swaddle can resemble the snug fit of the mother's womb; it is warm and your baby is contained. Being swaddled helps to inhibit the startle reflex previously mentioned in this book. Swaddling provides deep touch pressure and helps babies feel secure. A swaddled baby should be held or placed on his back—never on his tummy or side. When done correctly, swaddling is an effective technique to help calm your baby and to promote sleep. Swaddled babies are more settled and will usually sleep longer. If a baby is unsettled and it is not time for a feeding, try swaddling him. Sometimes it will calm him and get him organized, and sometimes it will help him fall asleep. If your baby does not seem to like swaddling, as demonstrated by him crying when you attempt it or arching away from it, try different times of the day, new ways to swaddle him (eg, 1 arm free, both arms free), or swaddle just the arms and leave the legs free to kick. You can also use different textured blankets that are softer, thinner, not so hot, etc, but don't give up! Some babies will tolerate being swaddled until about 9 to 12 weeks of age. However, if your baby starts to try to roll over before then, you should stop swaddling, because if your baby rolls over onto the stomach while swaddled, that is very dangerous. Because your baby's arms are swaddled, he can't push up on his arms to lift his head. It is best to swaddle fussy babies for all sleeps (day and night) and when they seem unsettled during awake times. Some babies also benefit from swaddling when they have trouble getting organized for feeding (see Chapter 10).

You don't need a special swaddle blanket for your newborn, but there are several swaddle blankets on the market ideal for swaddling. A light muslin or cotton blanket wrapped snugly around your baby works well too. These blankets are breathable, which prevents overheating. Sometimes swaddling will

Swaddling Safety Precautions

If your baby is attempting to roll over, swaddling is no longer a safe option, as she could roll over on to her tummy and not be able to lift her head up to breathe. Make sure her legs are not held straight and tightly wrapped, as this can lead to hip problems like dislocation or hip dysplasia. Avoid swaddling during her entire awake time, as she needs to move her arms and legs and explore her world.

change a baby's state of arousal (see Chapter 6). Now that you know about his states of arousal, use swaddling to change them. If fussy, swaddle to move him into quiet alert, and possibly to light sleep. If you find he sleeps too much when in a swaddle and is hard to wake up, swaddling may not a good option for him.

The typical way to swaddle is to place the blanket on a flat surface and turn down the top corner about 4 to 6 inches. Place your baby's head with his neck at the fold, so he is in the center of the blanket (Figure 12.24A). Next, pull one corner over and tuck it under your baby tightly (Figure 12.24B). It is preferred to move your baby's hands up near his mouth so he can suck on his fingers. Some parents move the arms down along the side or will start with 1 arm up and 1 arm down; it is up to you and what your baby likes best. Next, fold up the lower corner of the blanket over the shoulder (Figure 12.24C), and then wrap the other corner across his body and tuck the edge under him (Figure 12.24D). You can swaddle the baby with his knees bent or straight, but make sure the swaddle is not too tight and he can wiggle his hips. You can also swaddle so the baby's arms are under the blanket but the hands are near his mouth for self-soothing.

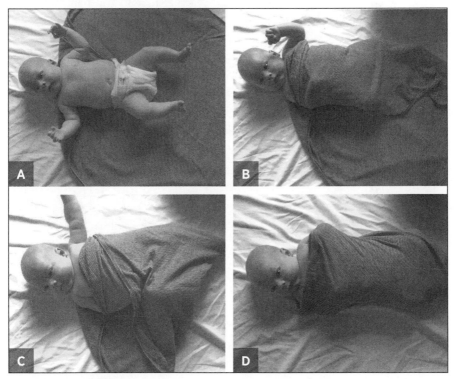

Figure 12.24. Swaddling.

Your Baby's Best Opportunities

Babies have a lot to learn in their first months, especially how to use their bodies to move and grow. The numerous ideas provided in this chapter help with your baby's development as well as decrease her fussiness. Give your baby the best opportunities to explore and use her limbs and muscles to develop coordination and become healthy and strong, as well as ways to calm, soothe, and keep her safe. Your baby will benefit in so many ways, and you will love watching it all happen!

> *"It is so exciting when your baby first lifts and moves her head from side to side during tummy time. She fussed at first but now is a tummy time champ! Because of all the tummy time, I think we are going to have an early crawler!"*
>
> Mother of a 3-month-old

Chapter 13

The Postpartum Family

Welcoming a new baby can trigger powerful emotions for both parents, from excitement and joy to fear, anxiety, or depression. Health care professionals do their best to educate you on a healthy pregnancy, help prepare for birth and delivery, and prepare you to leave the hospital with your new baby. Sometimes the reality of bringing home a baby can be challenging and emotionally draining. As much as we prepare for parenthood, it can be overwhelming at times, and you may worry when you feel unhappy or scared or have trouble coping with this huge change in your life. But there is help at hand, and you will feel well again!

Did You Know?

Many women will experience some mild mood changes during pregnancy and after the birth of their baby. Twenty percent will experience more significant symptoms of anxiety and depression. Women of every age, culture, race, and income level can develop perinatal mood and anxiety disorders. The transition to parenthood may be challenging, and mothers of fussy babies have a much higher risk for depression. There are effective treatment options to help you feel better again. The term *postpartum depression* is often used, but there are actually several forms of this illness that women may experience. With informed care you can prevent the worsening of any symptoms and fully recover. Remember, you are not alone, and you are not to blame!

The Baby Blues

Approximately 80% of women experience the "postpartum baby blues" after childbirth. The baby blues differ from postpartum depression in that the baby blues do not interfere with a new mother's ability to function in her everyday life. The baby blues start within the first few days after delivery and can last for up to 2 weeks. The symptoms pass quickly and do not have a lasting effect on the mother or the family. Because the baby blues are so common it is considered normal and not serious for the postpartum mother.

You may have the baby blues if you

- Feel sad or cry a lot.
- Feel moody or irritable.
- Have trouble sleeping, eating, or making decisions.
- Feel overwhelmed that you may not know how to take good care of your baby.
- Feel empty or lonely.
- Feel on edge or overly sensitive.
- Feel like you are not able to cope.
- Feel mentally or physically exhausted.

These feelings can be caused by some of the following:

- Changes in your body's hormones from the end of pregnancy and birth
- Unexpected physical discomfort
- Fatigue and sleep deprivation
- Expectations of your labor and delivery not realized
- Difficulty with breastfeeding

The baby blues usually go away on their own without treatment. Here's what you can do to help yourself.

- Get as much sleep as you can.
- Ask for help from your partner, family, and friends. Tell them exactly how they can help.
- Allow people you trust to help you with your baby.
- Take time for yourself and try not to feel guilty about needing some time away from the baby.
- Use the CALM method to help you understand your baby and gain confidence.

Postpartum Depression and Anxiety

Postpartum depression is different from the baby blues, as it is a clinical form of depression. This type of depression may be mistaken for baby blues at first, but the signs and symptoms are more intense and last longer. It can make it hard for a mother to take care of herself or her baby and handle other daily tasks. Symptoms usually appear within the first few weeks after the baby is born, but they can begin during pregnancy and up to a year after birth. Postpartum depression and/or anxiety is the most common complication after giving birth, and it is not a sign of weakness or being a "bad mother." Approximately 20% of postpartum women develop postpartum depression and 10% of postpartum women develop anxiety. They can experience them alone or combined. There's no single cause, and symptoms can range from mild to severe.

You may have postpartum depression if you

- Have feelings of anger or irritability.
- Have a lack of interest or difficulty bonding with your baby.
- Find yourself crying often and have feelings of sadness.
- Experience appetite or sleep disturbances.
- Have feelings of guilt, shame, and hopelessness about your mothering skills.
- Lose interest or pleasure in activities you used to enjoy.
- Have feelings of inadequacy as a mother.

Some of the reasons you may have postpartum depression include

- A personal history of depression or postpartum depression
- Anxieties about your ability to care for your baby
- Struggling with your sense of identity and feeling you've lost control over your life
- Infertility treatments, having multiples, or having a baby in the neonatal intensive care unit (NICU)
- Complications in your pregnancy, birth, or breastfeeding
- Marital or financial stress
- Premenstrual dysphoric disorder

"*My fussy baby increased my depression and anxiety, and I felt that added to baby's fussiness. Finding the right support group, a good therapist, medication, and a helping hand so I could get some sleep was so important. There is an indirect relationship between good sleep and depression for me!*"

Mother of 2 boys

You may have postpartum anxiety if you have

- Constant worry
- The feeling that something bad is going to happen
- Racing thoughts and the inability to sit still
- Appetite or sleep disturbances
- Panic attacks where you may feel shortness of breath, chest pain, dizziness, and tingling

Some of the reasons you may have postpartum anxiety include

- A personal history of anxiety or previous postpartum anxiety
- A thyroid imbalance

Receiving help promptly can help you manage your symptoms and allow you to feel supported and recover. The choice of treatment depends on how mild or severe your symptoms are. If you are able to fulfil your daily routine but your quality of life is affected, you may benefit from a postpartum support group or support counseling. If your postpartum depression and anxiety are preventing you from doing basic tasks, you should seek individual therapy to help you manage your symptoms. Your health care professional may also prescribe medications to help ease your symptoms quickly.

"*It was helpful for me to remember that stress begets stress. My fussy baby and my anxiety got in a feedback loop. The more she screamed, the more tense I got, and then she screamed more because she felt my physical stress. I had to break the loop. I would go for a walk, take a drive, call in support, put her in the crib, whatever it took.*"

Mother of 3 children

Postpartum Obsessive-Compulsive Disorder

Postpartum obsessive-compulsive disorder (OCD) is a type of postpartum anxiety disorder that affects 3% to 5% of new mothers. Its symptoms involve the mother's thoughts and behaviors, specifically toward her baby. It is characterized by repetitive thoughts or mental pictures, frequently about the baby being hurt. These intrusive thoughts can also be about germs, illness, or death of the mother herself or her baby. These thoughts can bring feelings of shame and guilt and can severely disrupt daily life. These mothers take actions to reduce their anxiety, such as taking the baby to the health care professional frequently because they are worried something is wrong. Others may avoid the stairs if they have obsessive thoughts about falling with the baby in their arms. Women with postpartum OCD are aware of these intrusive thoughts but are usually unable to control them. Research shows that although these thoughts and images are anxious in nature, they have a very low risk of being acted on.

You may have postpartum OCD if you have

- Obsessive thoughts (also known as intrusive thoughts) that are persistent and upsetting concerning a danger that involves your baby
- A sense of horror about these obsessions
- A fear of being left alone with your baby
- A fear of making poor decisions that may harm your baby
- Hypervigilance in trying to protect your baby
- Compulsions where you need to do something repeatedly to distract and reduce your fear

Some of the reasons you may have postpartum OCD include

- A personal history of anxiety or OCD
- Unmet expectations of motherhood that cause self-doubt and negative thoughts

This severe form of anxiety requires treatment to manage and control the symptoms. Postpartum OCD is temporary and treatable with professional help. Treatment options usually combine therapy and medication to fully manage the symptoms and help you cope. A qualified mental health professional can teach coping skills to improve your quality of life. There are several medication options designed to stop obsessive and compulsive thoughts from taking over and provide relief from the nervous energy and fears associated with postpartum OCD.

> "One of the most helpful things I realized in my post-partum support group is that intrusive thoughts are a manifestation of our fears, not our desires. It can be very scary when you're not sure where those ideas are coming from when they pop into your head and won't go away. Acknowledging that 'yes, that would be bad,' and then moving on is crucial."
>
> Mother of 2 children

Postpartum Post-traumatic Stress Disorder

Postpartum post-traumatic stress disorder (PTSD) has a distinct set of symptoms that set it apart from other postpartum mental health conditions. It develops out of a traumatic experience that took place before, during, or shortly after childbirth. This traumatic incident could have been real or perceived. It creates anxiety, as the flashbacks or memories to the event continually remind those with postpartum PTSD of the trauma they experienced. This is separate from postpartum depression but can co-occur. Overall, the 9% of women who develop postpartum PTSD after the birth of their baby feel as though they are in a constant state of distress, which causes physical, mental, emotional, and behavioral symptoms.

You may have postpartum PTSD if you have

- Flashbacks or nightmares related to pregnancy or birth
- Intrusive thoughts reexperiencing the real or perceived traumatic event
- Anxiety or panic attacks for seemingly no reason
- Irritability, difficulty sleeping, or hypervigilance
- Avoiding things that will trigger trauma, including thoughts, feelings, people, places, and details of an event
- Feeling a sense of detachment to those around you

Some of the reasons you may have postpartum PTSD include

- A history of PTSD symptoms from a past trauma
- A history of depression or anxiety
- Having an unplanned cesarean delivery
- A difficult, long, or painful delivery

• Feelings of lack of support and/or poor communication during your delivery

• Experiencing a severe physical complication related to the pregnancy or childbirth

• Your baby being placed in a NICU

Postpartum PTSD is highly treatable, and it is important to seek help as soon as the symptoms are identified. There are different therapies conducted by mental health care professionals that are highly effective helping you overcome fears, reduce stress, and bond with your baby. Many mothers who receive treatment for their trauma move on and do not experience reminders or flashbacks of the event again.

> "My husband was in the military overseas and was not able to be at the birth of our first child. I ended up have a C-section and I felt alone and scared. I attended a support group as well as took medication. I kept asking when I was not going to have to relive this experience and when would I not feel like this. I wanted to bond with my daughter, but I was unsure how to accomplish this. The group let me relive my experience until 1 day, I went to group and proudly told them that the cloud lifted and my postpartum PTSD was over. I was done with that experience. Years later I remember how much the trauma of my baby's birth affected my early months of motherhood. It was part of my journey."
>
> Mother of 2 children

Postpartum Psychosis

Postpartum psychosis is a rare, serious mood disorder that can develop suddenly after childbirth, usually within the first few weeks. It occurs in about 1 to 2 out of every 1,000 deliveries and has similar effects as a bipolar episode (manic-depressive episode). Women who experience psychosis have a break from reality, and the delusions and beliefs make sense to them. For this reason, postpartum psychosis is a very dangerous condition that can have tragic outcomes. Because of the risks, many women who experience postpartum psychosis are hospitalized while they wait for prescribed medication to take effect.

Someone with postpartum psychosis may

- Exhibit paranoia and suspiciousness.
- Have lost a sense of reality.
- Hallucinate (ie, seeing or hearing things that are not there).
- Have a decreased need for or inability to sleep.
- Have rapid mood swings or angry outbursts.
- Become confused or make poor decisions.
- Have trouble concentrating or remembering things.
- Show agitated or manic behavior.
- Have thoughts of harming herself or her baby.

Some of the reasons a woman may have postpartum psychosis include

- A history of previous postpartum psychosis
- A history of depression, anxiety, or OCD
- A personal or family history of bipolar disorder
- Having obsessive personality traits

Postpartum psychosis requires immediate attention. Women experiencing psychotic episodes almost always need hospitalization to protect the health and safety of both herself and her baby. There are antipsychotic medications, sedatives, and other mood-altering medications to control the psychosis. In addition to hospitalization and medication, women with postpartum psychosis can undergo psychotherapy with a mental health professional. With treatment, these women can make a full recovery and develop a healthy bond with their baby.

> *"I knew my wife was struggling with postpartum anxiety. Then one morning I knew something was different. She showed me a journal that she stayed up all night writing in on how to cure cancer. When I opened it, the whole journal was just scribbles. Then she told me how perfect our son was, and she would not let anyone do anything to make him less perfect. I was scared for my wife and my son. She was admitted to the hospital for 17 days. I am happy to report our son is now 9 years old and my wife is the best mother and I am so proud of her."*
>
> Father of 1 child

Postpartum Depression and Partners

Approximately 20% of new fathers and/or partners can experience paternal postpartum depression. It can begin during your partner's pregnancy or in the months afterward. Men who experience paternal postpartum depression may not understand how it developed; it is similar to postpartum depression in women. You may feel sad or fatigued, overwhelmed, or anxious, or have changes in your eating and sleeping patterns, similar to what mothers experience. This can have the same negative effects on the marital relationship and also affect bonding with your baby. Identifying the symptoms can help prevent you from suffering in silence. Half of all men who have a spouse experiencing postpartum depression will be depressed as well.

You may have postpartum depression if you

- Withdraw socially.
- Cannot focus on work and may feel generally distracted.
- Feel unmotivated, low energy, and fatigue.
- Become easily stressed and frustrated (anger outbursts).
- Have a change in sleep, weight, or appetite.
- Notice an onset of impulsive and risky behavior.

Some of the reasons you may have paternal postpartum depression include

- A continual lack of sleep
- A high-stress lifestyle, including family and career
- Relationship tensions with the mother or in-laws
- Feeling excluded from the bond between mother and baby
- Financial stress

Partners with paternal postpartum depression should be proactive in seeking help. It is important that you know you are not alone, you are not to blame, and you will feel well again with help. There is no shame in feeling depressed or anxious after the birth of your baby. It is a huge lifestyle change that can bring on emotional shifts. There are different medications, counseling from health care professionals, and support groups available to partners. Men can also participate in family-oriented groups to learn healthy coping and relationship skills. Similar to women, partners with paternal postpartum depression deserve recovery for themselves and their family.

> "It was our fourth child and I suddenly found myself avoiding being home and avoiding my newborn son. My wife was breastfeeding, and the baby would not take a bottle. With my 3 daughters I was always able to feed them with breast milk in a bottle. I felt left out, and I did not know how to comfort him because he would cry when I held him. My wife finally called me out; she told me that if I didn't know how to 'read' our baby, I would learn. So it was time. I took that advice and formed my own special bond with my son."
>
> Father of 4 children

Fussy Babies and Postpartum Depression

Fussy newborns can be especially challenging for parents already facing physical and mental exhaustion from caring for a new baby. Studies have observed that the more difficult it is to soothe the baby, the more distressed parents may be. Parents of highly irritable babies experience greater postpartum depression and/or anxiety symptoms. Caring for a baby with a difficult temperament takes an additional emotional toll, and having extra support and education may help you manage better. Learning about expected newborn behaviors and ways to calm a fussy baby, as we have learned throughout this book, can help you understand and care for your baby with greater confidence. Additional support may decrease the risk of postpartum depression and/or anxiety for you as well.

> "One of my favorite quotes is, 'Dogs bark; babies cry.' I've shared it with so many new moms at my stroller fitness classes. Babies cry; it's just what they do. You're not doing it wrong."
>
> Mother of 3 children

Finding Help and Support

If you are feeling depressed or anxious after your baby's birth, you may be reluctant or embarrassed to talk about it. If you are experiencing any symptoms of any of the postpartum mood disorders, anxiety, or the baby blues, it is important to call your health care professional. Don't wait and assume you will be able to handle it on your own; the sooner you seek help, the sooner you will feel—and function—better.

There are several reasons to believe that learning how to identify and dealing with infant crying behavior may be an effective way to improve the new parent confidence in his or her parenting abilities. Emerging evidence suggests it is beneficial to find ways of calming a baby as a strategy for treating postpartum depression and anxiety and the other perinatal mood disorders. A high-need baby demands so much attention and energy and can very easily drain your emotional and physical resources. Parents caring for babies with more difficult temperaments may need extra resources and education to help manage the emotional toll it can take. Early identification of baby fussiness may help identify parents with depressive symptoms in need of support. The advice I give to parents who are experiencing postpartum depression and a fussy baby is this: please take care of yourself and allow yourself some grace as you are all getting to know your new baby.

Here are additional ways to find support.

- Ask for support from your spouse/partner, family members, and friends.
- Find a local support group for new parents.
- Find a therapist or counselor who specializes in mood and anxiety disorders associated with pregnancy and childbirth.
- Accept offers of help from friends and family (eg, babysitting, cooking meals, cleaning).
- Make sleep a priority.
- Connect with a lactation consultant for any breastfeeding issues.
- Nourish yourself! Eat a healthy, well-balanced diet.
- Stay active and engage in healthy exercise when allowed.
- Use the CALM method to have a deeper understanding of your baby.

Without treatment, postpartum depression can make it harder to form strong bonds with your baby and the rest of your family. Postpartum depression or anxiety can cause emotional strain for everyone close to the family.

Here are some reasons to find help if you are experiencing any of the postpartum mood disorders.

- Fewer interactions with you baby, affecting you learning how to read your baby's cues
- Not being bothered by your baby's crying, thinking it's normal crying, and not responding accordingly
- Less motivation and energy to help your colicky baby
- Overreacting to your baby's crying due to low tolerance

Babies of mothers who have untreated postpartum depression are more likely to have sleeping and eating difficulties, excessive crying, and delays in language development.

> "OCD with intrusive thoughts—so fun—NOT! My postpartum support group, medication, and individual therapy saved my life and helped me through the super hard times. I learned to accept that it was OK to mourn my pre-mom life while starting a new chapter as a mom. I had found support and common ground with so many moms."
>
> Mother of 3 children

Some new parents may experience mild or manageable symptoms of the postpartum mood disorders; others may have a much harder time. This is a real illness, and you are not to blame. Don't wait and hope for improvement or try to carry it by yourself. You are not alone in your experiences, and there are people here to help you. Any new parent may become depressed or anxious during the pregnancy or up to a year after the birth of the baby; as many as 1 in 5 women have this experience during their lives. The information and tips in this book are a great way to gain insight on what to expect with crying babies and ways to help soothe them. Finding treatment and support helps you care for yourself and your baby and allows you to be the best parent you can be!

"I struggled with both postpartum depression and anxiety with 3 of my 4 children. I reached out, and with my husband's help and understanding, I was able to climb out of the darkness. I also joined a support group and gained so much insight from sharing my fears and feelings with family and trusted friends."

Stephanie Krantz, RN, BSN, IBCLC, PMH-C

Chapter 14

Beyond Colic: Disorders in Babies Older Than 6 Months

We hope you have read all the chapters focusing on the areas that may be related to your baby's fussiness; hopefully, you've gotten some answers that help you to understand your baby better. And we also hope you have identified some strategies that could work with your baby. Maybe life is going a little better for you and your baby. Or maybe the colic phase has passed and your baby is less fussy and has more regular sleep and feeding schedules; thus, caring for her is much easier.

But what if things aren't better and these problems persist past 6 months? What happens if your baby's irritability continues past the "normal" colic curve? To develop and thrive during the first year, a baby should be able to self-soothe and cope with the world around him. Most babies develop the skills to self-soothe and regulate behavioral states by 6 months of age. Prolonged problems with irritability, sleep, and feeding put a strain on parents and babies. You are exhausted, overwhelmed, and need some help! Fussiness or irritability is the most common trait with these older babies and toddlers.

In recent years, professionals from early childhood development have described difficulties with sleeping, feeding, irritability, self-soothing, temper tantrums, and mood regulation as *infant dysregulation* or *regulatory problems*. All infants have their own developmental progression, and every baby is different. These behaviors could be transient or intermittent, but some persist and increase to include more problems in the preschool years. We want to identify these difficulties as soon as possible so we can intervene early and help families when they are experiencing some of these behaviors. Some of these issues are early precursors to behavioral and cognitive problems later, so intervening early is best.

You are your baby's advocate, as she can't explain what she is feeling. You may be used to the lists of questions you receive at your well-baby visits; these usually are straightforward questions about your baby's general development, such as crawling, walking, and saying a few words. But for a deeper reflection of your baby's behavior the following considerations will help you to communicate these concerns with your primary care physician. Before your appointment, spend a few days focusing on your baby's behavior, organize your concerns, and take notes, so you can share them at the appointment. To help you with this process, the following outline lists behaviors we often see in older babies with continuing issues of crying, sleeping, and feeding behaviors as well as sensory processing issues.

1. What behaviors am I concerned about with my baby?
    - Clinginess; has difficulty separating from you
    - Irritability; cries a lot; acts unhappy and stressed much of the day
    - Can't calm down very well on his own; requires a lot of help from you to calm
    - Unsure of new people and new environments; is "painfully" shy
    - Does not transition well to different activities or different situations
    - Seems very rigid with routines and play activities
    - Shows defiance, temper tantrums, and aggressive behaviors; has unpredictable outbursts, sometimes for no reason, as seen by quickly escalating from being content to very irritable

2. What developmental milestones do you expect to see but have not seen yet?
    - *Language:* sounds, words, trying to communicate, frustration when he can't communicate his wants and needs, limited use of gestures to communicate (ie, reaching to be picked up, waving, clapping and pointing)
    - *Motor:* delayed milestones such as rolling, sitting, moving in and out of sitting, creeping, walking
    - *Play:* little interest in play or toys; relies on parent to entertain him; has a hard time initiating play on his own; no independent play skills
    - *Attention:* moves quickly from toy to toy; always moving, on the go, very active, difficulty sitting still to play
    - *Social:* limited interest in people; prefers objects; difficult to get your baby to look at you; rarely shows enjoyment with others

3. What concerns do I have about sleep? Be specific.
   - Won't fall asleep on her own
   - Needs extensive help to fall asleep; it takes longer than 30 minutes to place her to sleep
   - Won't nap or only takes catnaps
   - Extremely late bedtimes
   - Wakes more than 3 or 4 times at night to eat or to be calmed back to sleep
   - Nighttime awakenings lasting longer than 30 minutes
   - Depends on parental presence for sleep
   - Won't stay in the crib; eventually has to sleep with parent

4. What concerns do I have about feeding? Be specific.
   - Gags on food
   - Difficulty transitioning to pureed food and to table food, from breast to a bottle, or to a sippy or straw cup
   - Very picky with food; purses his lips, turns head and refuses
   - Prefers only 1 texture of foods (eg, only purees, only crunchy foods)
   - Prefers to drink liquids over eating solid foods
   - Strong dependence on breastfeeding, refusing solid foods
   - Won't sit in a high chair
   - Won't eat for anyone but mom
   - Needs a quiet, non-distracting environment to eat, or needs to be entertained during meal with toys, television, etc

5. What concerns do I have about my baby's ability to participate in caregiving routines and play that provide unwanted sensory experiences? Does he become more distressed with these activities than other children?
   - Resists daily care such as having his face and hands wiped, having hair washed, taking a bath, having his diaper changed, getting hands messy during feeding
   - Hates being restrained in a car seat, high chair, stroller, etc
   - Strongly dislikes tummy time
   - Fears movements such as being laid down for a diaper change, being passed off to another adult, rocking, or swinging
   - Startles easily to loud sounds or movements and takes a while to recover from the input

6. What behaviors do you see that seem unusual to you?
   - Rocking
   - Hand flapping
   - Head banging
   - High activity level; feels as if he is always moving
   - Is a risk-taker or a little daredevil, so is often unsafe
   - Tenses body; arching to avoid certain things, such as getting in the car seat or touching messy things

Your observations of these behaviors will help to identify if 1 of the following clinical disorders might be present. These disorders need to be taken seriously for 2 reasons. First, they cause significant stress and strain on the parent, the family, and the baby. Second, if these issues are left untreated and persist over a longer time, they can lead to developmental and behavioral problems in the toddler and preschool years. If several of these concerns are still apparent with your baby, a comprehensive evaluation is recommended.

Clinical Disorders

Many professionals in early childhood development attempt to find a classification system to help identify babies and toddlers with clinically impairing disorders and to avoid pathologizing children who are demonstrating possible "normal" variations of typical development. They also want to identify these babies and toddlers to provide them the intervention they need to improve long-term outcomes. In this chapter, we've outlined a few disorders that may be correlated to fussy babies who continue to be fussy beyond 6 months of age. This is by no means an exhaustive list of disorders, but it does identify some disorders that babies with a history of irritability may exhibit as they get a little older. This is also a basic overview of these disorders, so if you see some of these patterns in your baby or toddler, check out reliable resources to learn more about the specific disorders (see Resources).

One of these disorders is a *sensory processing disorder,* specifically *sensory over-responsivity disorder.* This disorder is often seen with infants and toddlers who continue to be irritable, who are often described as sensitive, and who cannot tolerate typical daily sensory experiences. We learned about all the sensory systems in Chapter 5, but what does having a sensory processing disorder mean? *Sensory processing* is the ability for an individual to take in sensory information from the world and interpret it to make appropriate motor and behavioral responses. Babies and toddlers who show exaggerated responses to sensory stimuli exhibit atypical responses such as overreacting when participating in typical roughhousing play with a parent or having difficulty tolerating simple daily care such as diaper changes or bath time. The may also overrespond to touch and bright lights. We also see that these babies don't always mouth toys for play, as typical babies do, and this often leads to difficulties with tolerating different food textures in their mouth, which affects their ability to transition to solid foods.

Feeding disorders are another clinical syndrome that may be associated with fussy babies or irritable toddlers. (See Chapter 10 for more information on feeding challenges.) There are many different types of feeding disorders. Your baby may have a feeding disorder of state regulation, which we learned about in Chapter 6. Feeding disorders can also include picky eating, difficulty transitioning to age-appropriate foods, or an undereating disorder, which usually is seen in babies or toddlers who lose weight or do not gain weight as expected by looking at the growth charts your pediatrician completes at each well-baby visit. Feeding disorders can be seen at any age.

Sleep disorders or sleep problems are seen sometimes in fussy babies and irritable toddlers. What is known about typical sleep in babies is that 90% of babies sleep through the night (ie, no breastfeeds, waking, or needing help to fall back asleep) by 10 months of age.

Sleep problems encompass a couple of different issues.

- *Sleep onset disorder* is seen when babies older than 6 months or toddlers take longer than 30 minutes to fall asleep, and this continues for more than 1 month.
- *Night waking disorder* is seen when babies awake multiple times during the night, as they often will breastfeed or need assistance to get back to sleep. They also prolong the time they are awake by wanting to play or eat. This disorder usually happens at 8 months or older and for more than 1 month.

Another disorder we see often with older toddlers is *overactivity disorder of toddlerhood*. With these toddlers we see a developmentally inappropriate activity level and impulsiveness compared with his peers. This includes things such as seeming to have excessive motor activity, having difficulty sitting still to play or to listen to books, and often being reported by parents that they are "on the go" all the time. They often have difficulty settling down for sleep and are often risk-takers or "little daredevils" who climb unsafely. This is typically identified in children from age 2 to 3 years.

A final disorder we sometimes see as fussy babies get older is *separation anxiety disorder*. This disorder is seen when babies or toddlers have excessive distress when they are separated from the primary caregiver, have difficulty separating to attend child care, or even become distressed when the parent just leaves the room. We can understand how this develops, as the fussy baby is so demanding and often demands attention primarily from his mother. The inability for the baby or toddler to separate totally affects his ability to separate for sleep. Keep in mind that some degree of separation anxiety continues to be normal for older babies and toddlers. However, when the level of distress exceeds what is expected for a child's age and developmental level, and it results in significant challenges for both parent and child, then it may be appropriate to explore if a separation anxiety disorder is present. When the symptoms last for more than 1 month and appear excessive or extreme, then it's possible that a disorder may be present.

There are many thoughts about how a regulatory problem should be categorized. Is it a medical diagnosis or an infant mental health diagnosis? Should we identify these regulatory problems as mild, moderate, or severe? Who do we treat, babies and toddlers with more moderate and severe issues, or could any family benefit from some intervention? Health care professionals used to take a wait and see approach in the hopes that the baby or toddler would just simply grow out of it. Thankfully, research has contributed to a better understanding of these patterns, and families are finally being listened to and receiving some help early on. The research is still evolving, but we are learning that when parents have concerns about their baby or toddler we should listen with clinical empathy and support and refer appropriately.

Which Professionals Are Involved?

There are a number of professionals who can assess your child to determine if he has one of these disorders. These professionals include developmental pediatricians, pediatric developmental psychologists, and occupational therapists. A comprehensive assessment by any of these professionals should include evaluating your baby or toddler by assessing their developmental performance, observing the problem behaviors, and doing an extensive parent interview to learn about the behaviors that are the causes of distress for parents and babies. This is much more comprehensive than a basic developmental assessment, which looks only at milestones of development. Occupational therapists also look more specifically at the sensory processing abilities of your baby.

Once the evaluation is completed, health care professionals determine the need for intervention as well as the type of intervention that is needed. Following is a brief overview of professionals who typically provide intervention and what their role is with infants and toddlers with these types of clinical disorders. Their roles overlap, so you most likely will not need to see all these professionals; however, sometimes a multidisciplinary approach is the best way to meet the needs of your family and baby. These professionals include

- *Occupational therapists* focus on developmental milestones, behavioral issues, feeding, sleep, play skills, and sensory processing.
- *Pediatric developmental psychologists* focus on behavioral issues and the parent-child relationship as well as developmental issues.
- *Infant mental health specialists* focus on social-emotional development and the parent-infant relationship.
- *Speech-language pathologists* focus on feeding skills as well as expressive and receptive language and communication deficits and social skills.

Finding the right professional to work with you and your family is critical for success. Not everyone has specific experience in treating babies and toddlers with sensory processing difficulties or crying, sleeping, and/or feeding difficulties, so you may need to ask questions about professionals' experience to be sure they have the type of expertise you require for the best chance of success for you and your baby.

Treatment Approaches

So what can we do for babies and toddlers who have these disorders? Early intervention is extremely important to increase the developmental potential. Accurate and early diagnosis can guide effective treatments before these patterns become set and more difficult to change. The right treatment will help you to understand your child better and help you make adjustments to her environment as needed to help her cope with her surroundings.

Treatment approaches may be more child focused or parent-child focused depending on the professional involved. The treatment will likely focus on support and reassurance for parents, parent education, sensory processing, and developmental tasks (motor, language, and play). Treatment may include some or all of the following: modifying daily routines, changing the environment, coaching parents on reading their baby's cues and understanding their baby's behaviors, developmental tasks, and sensory processing.

Left unaddressed, fussiness in older babies can lead to other problems later on. There may be more issues with sleep, feeding, language, emotions, ability to concentrate and learn, and relationships with family and others. A goal of intervening early is to enhance the capabilities of families to help their babies and toddlers develop, learn, and participate in the family. Through early identification and treatment of these disorders, it may be possible to prevent more serious, long-term problems in your child's sleep, feeding, attention/arousal, language, play, sensory processing, and emotional/behavioral difficulties in the future.

> *"My baby is turning a year old; it was a long year, but I really learned about the unique strengths he has. It took a while to get him to eat the foods that babies usually eat, to get him on a good sleep schedule, and to help him cope with the world around him, but now he is a star! I know we would be in a different place if we had not gotten occupational therapy services early in his life. He is now thriving at day care and is a happy little kid who enjoys playing with all his friends."*
>
> Mother of a 1 year old

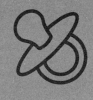

A CALMing Last Word

Patti Ideran, OTR/L, CEIM

As I worked on this book, I realized how much I wished this book was around to help me with our fussy baby! Written by experts who truly understand fussy babies and the difficulties they present, it is very comprehensive and gives you great insight into the complexities of having a fussy baby. We hope the solutions outlined in this book helped you along your journey. Having a fussy baby is not easy, and it is not just about a baby who cries a lot. There are many other factors that play a role. Our intent with this book was to educate you about those other aspects. Avoid advice that says your baby will grow out of it without offering the kind of help you need *now*.

The CALM Baby Method highlights all the key areas that will help you understand your baby. Interestingly, the things you learn in this book about sleep, sensory processing, arousal levels, feeding, motor development, and attachment are a foundation for your baby's formative years, and they apply to all developmental stages your baby will go through. Your baby may not cry and fuss as much when he gets older, but he communicates not only with verbal language but also his body language (or *cues*, as we introduced you to earlier). Earlier in the book we discussed how heredity and environment help your baby develop. This is good news, as you have total control over your baby's environment, now and in the future. So, when your baby is young, get her on the floor to play and engage in fun things, including tummy time, baby yoga poses, and massage.

We also took into consideration the mental health aspects of parenting a fussy baby, from attachment and bonding to postpartum depression. Don't think you can handle this all by yourself. Look for support from family, friends, support groups, and mental health professionals. You need to take care of yourself so you can take care of your baby and family. Eat healthy, meditate, or exercise. Bottom line: give yourself a well-deserved break!

Having children is a gratifying experience, but it's not always easy or fun! The fussy time is difficult, but you will get through it. Something more enjoyable is on the horizon (and then you hit the tween years, which is a whole other book!). Being a parent is a learning process, as is being a baby! It's new to both of you. Even if you have been here before, every baby is different. As a parent you will go through ups and downs, highs and lows, but just remember to always reach out to resources like this book and others about the age and stage you're going through. Hopefully, the CALM Baby Method has given you some solutions for those fussy days and sleepless nights and has helped bring more smiles than tears to you and your baby.

Resources

Recommended Parenting Books and Articles

Bennett SS, Indman P. *Beyond the Blues: Understanding and Treating Prenatal and Postpartum Depression & Anxiety.* Untreed Reads; 2019
Contains the most current pregnancy and postpartum resources for prevention and treatment of mental health challenges for all parents. Updated information and research about medications, as well as complementary and alternative options, are included. Direct and compassionate, it is required reading for those experience postpartum depression before or after the baby is born and for all professionals working with them.

Damian LA, Johnson K. Nipple flow rates: what are they really and how does this affect our clinical practice? Dr Brown's Medical. Accessed August 2, 2020. https://www.drbrownsbaby.com/medical/wp-content/uploads/2016/08/DBM-MilkFlowRates-Dayton-Article.pdf
This article describes nipple flow rates and compares the variability based on a research study.

Enten E. Over-diagnosed and over-prescribed. The Doctor Will See You Now. Published November 12, 2011. Accessed August 2, 2020. www.thedoctorwillseeyounow.com/content/kids/art3497.html
A pediatrician's explanation of the differences between colic and acid reflux in babies and suggested treatment approaches.

Faure M. *The Baby Sense Secret: Learn How to Understand Your Baby's Moods for Happy Days and Peaceful Nights.* DK; 2010
Written by an occupational therapist, this is a definite go-to baby book for new parents. It describes your baby's first year after birth and discusses sensory and motor development, sleep, and social-emotional

development, as well as your baby's personality. It is packed with suggestions on how to get through the first year. It helps parents understand their baby and their own feelings as a parent of a young baby.

Garabedian H. *Itsy Bitsy Yoga: Poses to Help Your Baby Sleep Longer, Digest Better, and Grow Stronger.* Simon & Schuster; 2004
This is a fun book that offers a wide variety of fun movement and positive touch experiences for babies and parents that help with bonding, attachment, and motor and sensory development.

Heath A, Bainbridge N. *Baby Massage: The Calming Power of Touch.* DK Publishing Inc; 2004
We love the pictures in this book showing all the different massage strokes. It teaches you the benefits of baby massage as well as all the massage strokes.

Kleiman K. *The Postpartum Husband: Practical Solutions for Living With Postpartum Depression.* Xlibris Corp; 2000
This hands-on guide includes straightforward, supportive information and specific recommendations to help partners deal with the effect of depression after the birth of a baby.

McClure V. *Infant Massage: A Handbook for Loving Parents.* 4th ed. Bantam Books; 2017
This book is the gold standard in infant massage, written by the founder of Infant Massage USA. It educates you about the benefits of massage as well as the powerful effects of positive touch experiences.

Nugent K. *Your Baby Is Speaking to You: A Visual Guide to the Amazing Behaviors of Your Newborn and Growing Baby.* Houghton Mifflin Harcourt Publishing Co; 2011
Beautiful pictures of babies highlight this book, illustrating your baby's subtle cues and what they mean.

Ripton N, Potock M. *Baby Self-feeding: Solid Food Solutions to Create Lifelong, Healthy Eating Habits.* Fair Winds Press; 2016
This book is written by a feeding specialist and reviews the basics of feeding with a special focus on transitions to solid foods.

Satter E. *Child of Mine: Feeding With Love and Good Sense.* Bull Publishing Co; 2000
A warm, supportive, and entertaining book for parents about basic nutrition for infants and young children. It provides a professional nutrition reference on topics such as breastfeeding, bottle-feeding, starting table foods, feeding schedules, healthy snack ideas, and more.

Siegel DJ, Hartzell M. *Parenting From the Inside Out: How a Deeper Self-understanding Can Help You Raise Children Who Thrive.* 10th anniversary ed. Penguin Group; 2014
If you are a parent who wants to gain more insight into how your childhood experiences might shape your approach to parenting, this is a great read with many healing and positive messages as well as interesting scientific findings.

Turgeon H, Wright J. *The Happy Sleeper: The Science-Backed Guide to Helping Your Baby Get a Good Night's Sleep—Newborn to School Age.* Penguin Group; 2014
This is a great resource about the importance of sleep and how to work on good sleep at different stages.

VandenBerg KA, Hanson MJ. *Coming Home from the NICU: A Guide for Supporting Families in Early Infant Care and Development.* Paul H. Brookes Publishing Co; 2013
This is a fabulous resource for parents who had a premature baby who spent any time in the neonatal intensive care unit (NICU). It has practical information to help you with the transition to home and life with your sensitive baby.

Zachry AH. *Retro Baby: Cut Back on All the Gear and Boost Your Baby's Development With More Than 100 Time-tested Activities.* American Academy of Pediatrics; 2014
In the new world of a lot of baby equipment and too much technology, this is an excellent resource to bring you back to the basics of playtime with your baby. It educates you about the risks of some of the new baby equipment as well as the effects of overexposure to too much technology.

Recommended Websites

Baby Center

https://www.babycenter.com

This website's advisory board includes experts in all areas of pediatric care, including physicians, psychologists, registered nurses, and dietitians. It hosts numerous up-to-date articles on a variety of baby topics from pregnancy, babies, toddlers, and preschoolers to big kids (aged 5–8 years). There is a tracker for your baby's development.

ChildLight Education Company

https://www.childlightyoga.com

This is a website where you can sign up for training as a yoga teacher, as well as some e-learning courses for families. It also has a directory of certified teachers in pediatric yoga.

EatRight.org

https://www.eatright.org

This website, from the Academy of Nutrition and Dietetics, is a professional nutrition resource center. EatRight.org provides tips on food safety, food label reading, breastfeeding basics, what to feed your infants and young children, and more. The website contains articles, tips, videos, and tools that you can use to help provide a healthy diet to your entire family.

Ellyn Satter Institute

https://www.ellynsatterinstitute.org

A nonprofit organization's team of dieticians, nutritionists, and educators provides parents with information and guidance to work on mealtimes and feeding concerns.

Feeding Flock

https://www.feedingflock.com/tools

This website, authored by a group of nursing and feeding experts, gives parents and professionals a wealth of information about screening children for feeding problems.

HealthyChildren.org

https://www.healthychildren.org

This site is an excellent resource for parents about anything related to children's health. As the official American Academy of Pediatrics (AAP) website for parents, it has the most current research by expert pediatricians. The AAP mission is to ensure optimal physical, mental, and social health and well-being for all infants, children, adolescents, and young adults.

Infant Massage USA

https://www.infantmassageusa.org

Infant Massage USA is an organization that trains professionals to become certified educators of infant massage. It also teaches parents about the benefits of infant massage and has an educator directory to help you find a class in your area.

International Hip Dysplasia Institute

https://hipdysplasia.org

This excellent site educates about hip dysplasia and its prevention. It has a medical advisory board of pediatric orthopedic surgeons from around the world. They have a wealth of information about safe swaddling, baby wearing, and baby carriers. They also rate "hip healthy" products and provide links to the companies that make the products.

Pathways.org

https://pathways.org

This is a great website for learning about typical milestones in development. The advisory board comprises experts in the fields of pediatric medicine and occupational, speech, and physical therapy. It has activities and resources by age of your baby. Its focus is to help maximize your baby's potential, and it helps you keep them on track and catch potential developmental delays.

Pediatric Sleep Council

https://www.babysleep.com

This is a great website that offers expert advice from leaders in the field of pediatric sleep, including psychologists and physicians. It offers information on a variety of sleep topics, including age-by-age sleep advice. Just type in a question and they respond with a variety of expert opinions on the topic.

Postpartum Dads

www.postpartumdads.org

The Postpartum Dads website was created by PSI Dad's Coordinator David Klinker as a forum to help dads and families by providing firsthand information and guidance through the experience of perinatal mood disorders.

Postpartum Support International

https://www.postpartum.net

Postpartum Support International is dedicated to helping families experiencing postpartum depression, anxiety, and distress. The organization wants you to remember that you are not alone, you are not to blame, and with help you can heal.

Sensory Processing Disorder Foundation

https://www.spdfoundation.net

As a leader in sensory processing disorder research and education, this is a valuable website to learn about sensory processing disorders. Its emphasis is clearly more oriented to the preschooler and school-aged child; however, it has great descriptions about what sensory processing disorder is as well as checklists and red flags to identify disorders in all ages.

Zero to Three

https://www.zerotothree.org

Zero to Three is a fabulous organization that has the most updated information about policy and advocacy for young children. It is an excellent resource for professionals and parents to ensure all babies and toddlers have a strong start in life. They have information about early learning, early development, and skills for parents of infants and children 0 to 3 years old.

Behavior Diary

The Behavior Diary discussed in Chapter 3 is on the following page and is a blank version for your own use. With this diary we look at and keep track of the 5 behaviors that your baby exhibits: sleeping, eating, crying, fussing, and awake times. Complete this diary for 3 to 5 days, which will allow you to determine if there is a pattern to these behaviors. Refer to Chapter 3 for more information.

BEHAVIOR DIARY

DAY 1 _/_/_

AM	Midnight	12:15 AM	12:30 AM	12:45 AM	1:00 AM	1:15 AM	1:30 AM	1:45 AM	2:00 AM	2:15 AM	2:30 AM	2:45 AM	3:00 AM	3:15 AM	3:30 AM	3:45 AM	4:00 AM	4:15 AM	4:30 AM	4:45 AM	5:00 AM	5:15 AM	5:30 AM	5:45 AM
AM	6:00 AM	6:15 AM	6:30 AM	6:45 AM	7:00 AM	7:15 AM	7:30 AM	7:45 AM	8:00 AM	8:15 AM	8:30 AM	8:45 AM	9:00 AM	9:15 AM	9:30 AM	9:45 AM	10:00 AM	10:15 AM	10:30 AM	10:45 AM	11:00 AM	11:15 AM	11:30 AM	11:45 AM
PM	Noon	12:15 PM	12:30 PM	12:45 PM	1:00 PM	1:15 PM	1:30 PM	1:45 PM	2:00 PM	2:15 PM	2:30 PM	2:45 PM	3:00 PM	3:15 PM	3:30 PM	3:45 PM	4:00 PM	4:15 PM	4:30 PM	4:45 PM	5:00 PM	5:15 PM	5:30 PM	5:45 PM
PM	6:00 PM	6:15 PM	6:30 PM	6:45 PM	7:00 PM	7:15 PM	7:30 PM	7:45 PM	8:00 PM	8:15 PM	8:30 PM	8:45 PM	9:00 PM	9:15 PM	9:30 PM	9:45 PM	10:00 PM	10:15 PM	10:30 PM	10:45 PM	11:00 PM	11:15 PM	11:30 PM	11:45 PM

DAY 2 _/_/_

AM	Midnight	12:15 AM	12:30 AM	12:45 AM	1:00 AM	1:15 AM	1:30 AM	1:45 AM	2:00 AM	2:15 AM	2:30 AM	2:45 AM	3:00 AM	3:15 AM	3:30 AM	3:45 AM	4:00 AM	4:15 AM	4:30 AM	4:45 AM	5:00 AM	5:15 AM	5:30 AM	5:45 AM
AM	6:00 AM	6:15 AM	6:30 AM	6:45 AM	7:00 AM	7:15 AM	7:30 AM	7:45 AM	8:00 AM	8:15 AM	8:30 AM	8:45 AM	9:00 AM	9:15 AM	9:30 AM	9:45 AM	10:00 AM	10:15 AM	10:30 AM	10:45 AM	11:00 AM	11:15 AM	11:30 AM	11:45 AM
PM	Noon	12:15 PM	12:30 PM	12:45 PM	1:00 PM	1:15 PM	1:30 PM	1:45 PM	2:00 PM	2:15 PM	2:30 PM	2:45 PM	3:00 PM	3:15 PM	3:30 PM	3:45 PM	4:00 PM	4:15 PM	4:30 PM	4:45 PM	5:00 PM	5:15 PM	5:30 PM	5:45 PM
PM	6:00 PM	6:15 PM	6:30 PM	6:45 PM	7:00 PM	7:15 PM	7:30 PM	7:45 PM	8:00 PM	8:15 PM	8:30 PM	8:45 PM	9:00 PM	9:15 PM	9:30 PM	9:45 PM	10:00 PM	10:15 PM	10:30 PM	10:45 PM	11:00 PM	11:15 PM	11:30 PM	11:45 PM

DAY 3 _/_/_

AM	Midnight	12:15 AM	12:30 AM	12:45 AM	1:00 AM	1:15 AM	1:30 AM	1:45 AM	2:00 AM	2:15 AM	2:30 AM	2:45 AM	3:00 AM	3:15 AM	3:30 AM	3:45 AM	4:00 AM	4:15 AM	4:30 AM	4:45 AM	5:00 AM	5:15 AM	5:30 AM	5:45 AM
AM	6:00 AM	6:15 AM	6:30 AM	6:45 AM	7:00 AM	7:15 AM	7:30 AM	7:45 AM	8:00 AM	8:15 AM	8:30 AM	8:45 AM	9:00 AM	9:15 AM	9:30 AM	9:45 AM	10:00 AM	10:15 AM	10:30 AM	10:45 AM	11:00 AM	11:15 AM	11:30 AM	11:45 AM
PM	Noon	12:15 PM	12:30 PM	12:45 PM	1:00 PM	1:15 PM	1:30 PM	1:45 PM	2:00 PM	2:15 PM	2:30 PM	2:45 PM	3:00 PM	3:15 PM	3:30 PM	3:45 PM	4:00 PM	4:15 PM	4:30 PM	4:45 PM	5:00 PM	5:15 PM	5:30 PM	5:45 PM
PM	6:00 PM	6:15 PM	6:30 PM	6:45 PM	7:00 PM	7:15 PM	7:30 PM	7:45 PM	8:00 PM	8:15 PM	8:30 PM	8:45 PM	9:00 PM	9:15 PM	9:30 PM	9:45 PM	10:00 PM	10:15 PM	10:30 PM	10:45 PM	11:00 PM	11:15 PM	11:30 PM	11:45 PM

Baby Behavior
S = sleeping E = eating C = crying F = fussing A = awake (content)

Growth Charts

As described in Chapter 2, the following are 4 examples of growth charts for an infant boy and an infant girl 0 to 24 months of age (regarding length, weight, and head circumference).

Birth to 24 months: Boys
Head circumference-for-age and
Weight-for-length percentiles

NAME _____

RECORD # _____

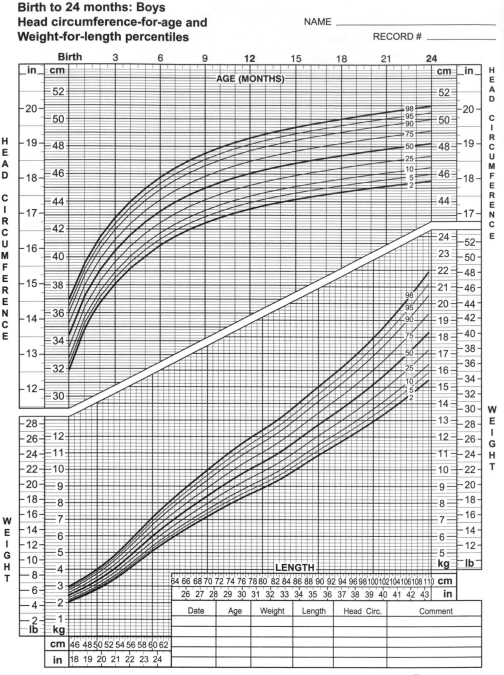

Published by the Centers for Disease Control and Prevention, November 1, 2009
SOURCE: WHO Child Growth Standards (http://www.who.int/childgrowth/en)

Birth to 24 months: Boys
Length-for-age and Weight-for-age percentiles

NAME _____

RECORD # _____

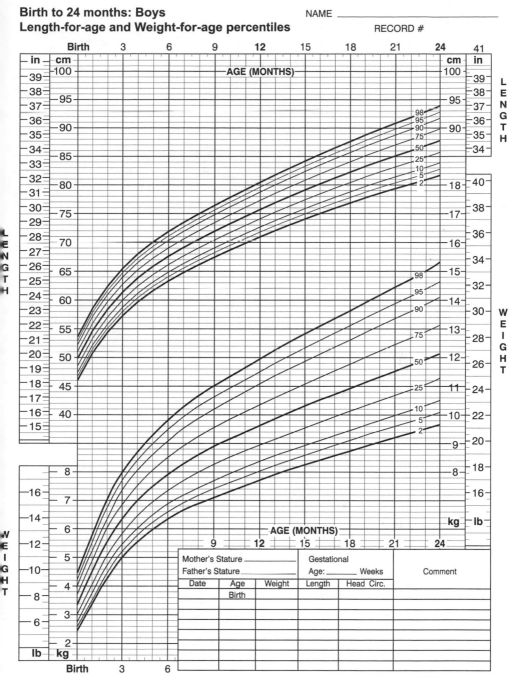

Mother's Stature _____			Gestational	
Father's Stature _____			Age: _____ Weeks	Comment
Date	Age	Weight	Length	Head Circ.
Birth				

Published by the Centers for Disease Control and Prevention, November 1, 2009
SOURCE: WHO Child Growth Standards (http://www.who.int/childgrowth/en)

SAFER · HEALTHIER · PEOPLE™

CDC

Birth to 24 months: Girls
Head circumference-for-age and
Weight-for-length percentiles

NAME _____

RECORD # _____

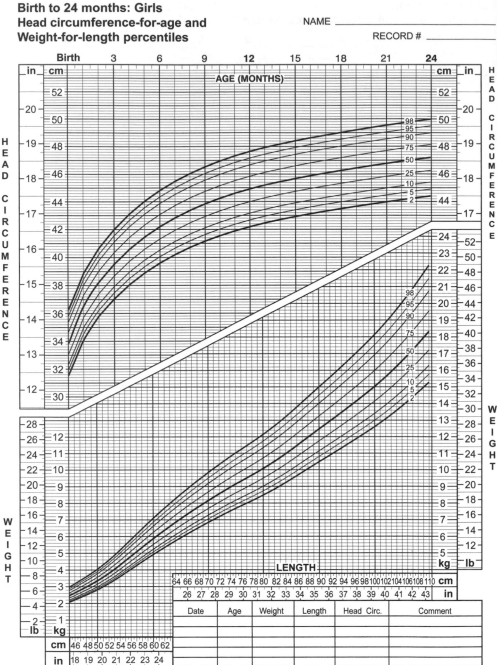

Published by the Centers for Disease Control and Prevention, November 1, 2009
SOURCE: WHO Child Growth Standards (http://www.who.int/childgrowth/en)

Birth to 24 months: Girls
Length-for-age and Weight-for-age percentiles

NAME _____

RECORD # _____

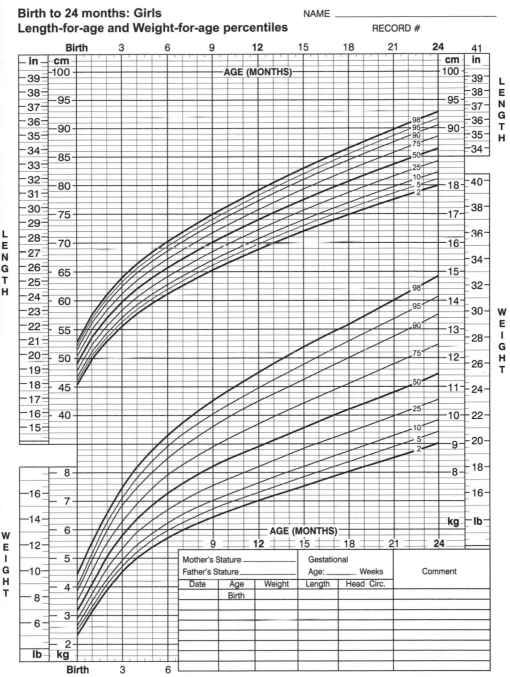

Index